HIPPOS EAT GRASS

HIPPOS EAT GRASS

Busting the Fat Myth

Odyle Knight

HIPPOS EAT GRASS
Busting the Fat Myth

@Copyright Odyle Knight 2011
ISBN 978-0-9805628-1-1

Also by Odyle Knight

BALI MOON
A Spiritual Odyssey

BALI MAGIC
Reflections of a Reluctant Psychic

odyleknight@hotmail.com
www.odyleknight.weebly.com

Cover design by Maria Thezar
Illustrations adapted by Carla Ball

CONTENTS

This book is dedicated to every person who has ever felt diminished because of the perceived way they look but innately believes in the perfection of creation, and in themselves as part of that divine plan. You were born beautiful, both on the inside and out, and in beauty you will always remain. So be true to yourself and the universe and live an authentic, valuable life.

Acknowledgements

To all those many people who have inspired me to write this book with your tales of courage, insight and ultimate strength I thank you for sharing your journey so that others will not feel alone and lost on theirs.

To the luminous Venus triangle of female energy that spanned continents, you are all part of a universal plan to bring love and light into a world that has lost its way by diminishing the beauty of all life. Sally you are my rock, Carla, the arrow to carry my vision into the wind, and lovely Cheryl, a channel of positive energy and optimism. Thanks to Richard for his astute editorial slant, Sarah for her guidance and friendship, Judy and Sue for their welcome input and the talented Maria for her artistic gift.

To the cosmic forces that helped shape this book, I thank you for your direction and resolve in insisting that beauty in all its forms be acknowledged and prized. As part of a universal plan, we are all perfect in our own right.

THE LAW OF THE JUNGLE

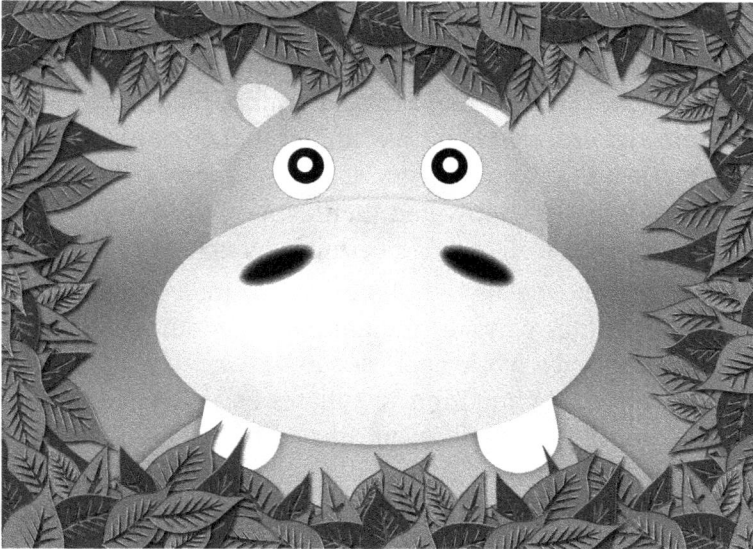

Have you ever been held captive in a jungle hut by a masticating rhino when you're dying to have a pee? I have, in Nepal. I went to Nepal on the advice of an old fortune teller who I chanced upon on the steps of the Royal Palace in Bangkok. As he gazed at my palm, he uttered the fateful words. 'The road to your destiny leads from Bombay.'

Not one to question the advice of a wise old fortune teller, especially one perched on golden palace steps, I set off in search of it. My destiny. Along the way I took in the frantic sights, smells, colors of India looking for clues. None came, until I crossed the border into Nepal. After an arduous journey along one of the most treacherous roads in the world that wound precariously around the Himalayas, my rickety bus stopped at a small dusty village. After a bumpy jeep ride along an overgrown track I reached a ring of thatched huts.

That's how I came to be in the jungle of Nepal, held hostage by a rhino. The toilet block lay some twenty feet away from my hut but there was no way I was making a run for it in the dark. The rhino, oblivious to my concerns, munched away happily on the grass outside. Trapped, I spent the night listening to it chomping grass and trying not to inhale the rhino's hot breath through the hut's log walls.

Lying awake on the bed with nothing better to do, I had a revelation. Here was this huge rotund animal just inches away. All night it chewed and ground grass and crunched some more. A big brute of a beast that lived on grass, with perhaps a few plants and berries thrown in every now and then. Not only did it have a frugal diet, it also chewed well. I could certainly vouch for that.

So how come it was fat? According to man's theory that food x exercise = weight, why has the animal kingdom got it so wrong? Rhinos can certainly work up a sweat and they basically eat only grass, as do elephants and hippos. Whales live on small crustaceans called krill but they are still a big bag of blubber. And what about snakes? A python can devour a whole squawking pig or goat in one gulp but I've never seen a fat snake. Despite their greed, they remain slithery.

The reason I know rhinos work up a sweat is that I already had an unfortunate encounter with one. It happened on my first day in the lodge when I set out on a jungle walk. As the ranger guided me along the scrub path, the ground rumbled like a subterranean earthquake and I heard a mighty clash. I stood rooted to the spot while the guide started to sweat. It was not a good sign so I began to sweat too. Then he darted off for a closer look.

Was he kidding? Leaving me alone while the earth grumbled all around me. I thought it was about to open up and swallow me. Then came another mighty bang and then another. The ranger ran back over to my side and muttered, 'Two rhinos fighting. Quick, run and hide behind a tree!' he added, before disappearing among some bushes.

Now he really had me in a panic. I looked for cover but the only trees scattered around me had trunks the size of my wrist. This was obviously virgin forest, with newly planted saplings all around. Did he really think my ample body was going to be concealed behind one of those spindly poles? With no other choice I quickly ran behind one, trying to squash my breasts so they wouldn't give me away.

All of a sudden the earth trembled and a rampaging rhino thundered past me, missing me by a hair's breadth. I was petrified, cast in stone. The guide led my shaking self back to the camp. 'The next time you see a charging rhino,' he advised, 'run zigzag. A rhino's head is so heavy it can't turn its neck fast enough to keep track of you.'

The guide was whistling into the wind. There wasn't going to be a next time because I was about to lock myself in the cabin and not come out for the next two days. Besides, what made him think I could escape a rampaging rhino under any condition? I was the delicate type, not marathon woman. I was no sportswoman but rather an artistic sort who would much rather paint a rhino than try to outrun one.

I'm also weak willed when it comes to food so the smell of toasting marshmallows at the camp fire that evening finally induced me to emerge. I'm glad I did. Around the campfire with all the guests wistfully singing John Denver songs and with me joining in for 'Leaving on a Jet Plane', preparing my retreat and foregoing my destiny, that's when it happened.

He walked into the circle, the head of the camp in his jungle greens. Nepal's answer to Pierce Brosnan. The fire sparked as soon as our eyes met. When we went for a stroll later on that night there was magic all around, as moonlight filtered through the canopy of leaves. Serenaded by a chorus of crickets, it was sheer bliss. The two of us under a star filled night that frosted the sky with sherbet.

Had it registered at the time that a prowling bear could have pounced on us or a lethal boa constrictor could have slid out from the bushes, or that the rhino would return to finish me off, well it might have dented the magic of the moment. But only a little. So I decided to stay in the jungle, on and off for the next two years.

It was not only my fascination with the man that kept me there but also the allure of the jungle. There was so much to learn from the animals and over time I came to understand the laws of nature a little better. Each species was unique in its own right and each looked and behaved differently. That was what made them special.

Most feared by the rangers was an encounter with a bear in the bushes because their instinct was to attack. Rhinos came next because most have a mean temper and with a ton of metal charging at you, look out! With several nasty gorings in the past they were taking no chances. However with a rhino, there was a chance it would bolt away. I had yet to spot an elusive tiger but had crossed paths with a sleepy leopard that didn't seem to be either aroused or offended by my presence.

My favorite was the elephants. They are the largest land animals on earth but also one of the gentlest. Each morning I awoke to the sound of the elephants heralding in the start of a brand new day. There were nine elephants in the stables and they trumpeted happily at the crack of dawn. They rejoiced in life and the bliss of the moment and appeared to be the happiest of beasts.

Elephants like to have a good time. Each night after all the guests had gone to sleep, we would creep into the elephant compound and sit in silence to watch their antics. Under a big bright moon, the elephants danced and sang and crooned. They threw hay around with gay abandon until they had stacks piled on their head and poking out from behind their ears or wrapped around their waists like a huge hula skirt. Together they would sway and sway and warble to each other.

We resisted the urge to laugh because elephants are sensitive and their feelings are easily hurt. You don't want to offend an elephant. One day an elephant took exception to one of the drivers. The foolish man was ordering him around and overloading him with hay. With one whack of his trunk, the annoyed elephant knocked him over and knelt on him. End of story. As I said, you don't want to offend an elephant.

Still these huge animals can be the most playful of creatures, with a delightful sense of humor. I watched one day as a cat that hitched a ride into the jungle on the back of a jeep ran mischievously between one of the elephant's legs. The elephant watched the cat's antics patiently and then with perfect precision gathered up a batch of hay with her trunk and then spat it out, burying the cat under it. The cat emerged unharmed but learnt not to mess with an elephant in the future.

Elephants also love the water. Most days I would go down to the creek and play right alongside them. One of the keepers encouraged me to get up onto docile Ana's back, who was the sweetest of all. I hated having to step on her leg to do so. Ana looked me in the eye with her long sumptuous lashes and smiled. When I felt her soft flesh squelch under mine we bonded. Once I was on up her back, she flopped down in the creek and showered me with trunk loads of water. Bliss.

Such is the essence of the animal kingdom. Animals come in all shapes and sizes. They come in splendid packages, equally beautiful and fascinating. Each has its own temper, mood and eccentricities. None is more captivating than the other and each has an integral part to play. That variety makes up life and we prize it.

Why then do we not afford the same honor and dignity to people? There is uniqueness in every person and in every creation, just as there is in animals. Our failure to recognize it is the reason why I wrote this book. It's time we realized we are all part of a greater plan and that we are each stunning and special in our own right.

Modern society pressures us to conform to some dreadful cookie cutter shape, based on the premise that the original package is defective, unworthy or imperfect in some way. It demands that large people be whittled down like some thick plank of wood or cast aside like driftwood on some deserted beach. As if being more is less.

An elephant would never stand for it, for it is far too proud and regal. In fact it would pound the perpetrator into the ground, as would a rhino or a hippo. A whale would swallow you whole. It's an affront to every person on the planet to suggest that we should be any less than we are, at OUR personal best. It is also an insult to the perfection of God's work and the intelligence of the universe. We are perfect just as we were born to be and at our best exactly as we were intended.

P.S I was the chubbiest girl in the jungle and I got the man!
…Why don't they ever show that in Hollywood?

ALL CREATURES GREAT AND SMALL

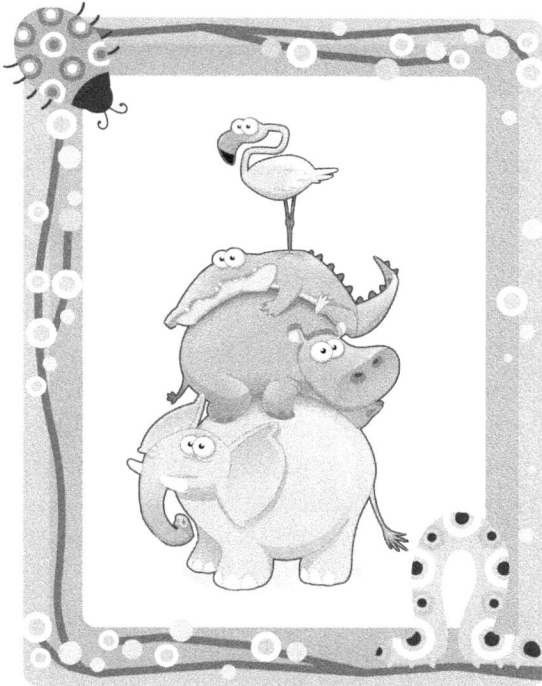

Now I ask you. When Noah was receiving instructions from God on how to save the world by building an ark and taking on board two of every animal species, did God discriminate? Did he say leave the fat ones behind? Did he ask them each to step on a scale to decide whether they were worth saving or send off the fatties to shed a few pounds before they could board, claiming they'd sink the boat?

Did he blame them for every ill that had befallen the world or insist they had caused the flood by peeing more than the rest or by chomping up the earth's resources with their voracious appetite? No,

God did not judge but instead loved them all equally because they were each his creation, perfect in their own right.

It's a curious thing that most species in the animal kingdom are chubby or at least a little bit fleshy. It may be a survival thing. All those hours spent chewing on those bamboo poles have done pandas no favors weight wise. Boy are they cute, though. Then there are koalas, bison, yaks, sheep and bears, raccoons, armadillos, rabbits, badgers, wombats, otters and seals. Pigeons, owls and chickens are chunky under all their feathers and even little sparrows are round.

The leaner animals are not necessarily the most likeable. In fact most are hard to take to. Snakes, praying mantis and stick insects are not an endearing lot. The rangier ones include among their ranks dingoes, hyenas, feral dogs and goats. They all look like they need a good feed and make the strangest sounds. No they're definitely not an appealing bunch and not the type you'd choose to keep as pets.

In case you're wondering what the heaviest animal on the planet is, the whale weighs in at number one. The blue whale tops the list at a massive 400,000 pounds. How they managed to pop one onto a scale is beyond me and what manner of scales could carry that amount of weight? Is that their weight on land or at sea because water flotation could help them drop a few pounds? If I was a whale I would insist on an aquatic weigh in so I could appear more buoyant. If you have any doubts about the sincerity of a whale, their heart alone weighs an amazing 2000lbs so there's a whole lot of loving going on.

Now here's an interesting fact you can pop into the conversation when you're sitting dejected at a party, starved of any real conversation or food. A pang of conscience has forced you to forgo the pleasures of the appetizer tray in favor of a tepid glass of Evian water and you whimper as you watch your thin party friends demolish the French Onion dip and saltine crackers. Cough loudly and then interject.

'Don't you think it's oddly poetic,' you offer, 'that no other mammal on earth is two steps above microscopic in the food chain and it happens to be the largest animal on the planet? A whale eats small crustaceans no bigger than your little finger, *krill a*ctually,' you add, sounding very worldly as you hold up your pinkie to illustrate. 'What's more,' you state loudly, as you go in for the kill, 'the blue whale only eats during the polar summer feeding season. The rest of the year, for eight months of it in fact, the whale doesn't eat anything at all!'

Strangely the whale lives off its stored fat during that time but I recommend you don't mention it in case some vicious skinny suggests you do the same. If any one of your party friends looks unimpressed by your brilliant expose, throw this in while you're at it. 'Even though we weren't around to see what dinosaurs ate, scientists acknowledge that many of their kind were herbivores. How come a whale stays fat while it's starved for most of the year and the dinosaur got so hefty living off a patch of cabbages or a bunch of shredded leaves? How come?'

Of course no one will be able to come up with a reasonable answer so you can feel vindicated when you go in for the main course of pate de foie gras in aspic. Make sure you put a generous serving of potato salad on the side to make up for it and an extra helping of crème caramel with a great dollop of cream for added effect!

Coming in as second on the heavy animal list is the largest of all land mammals, the African elephant at 11,000 pounds and its cousin the Indian species at 8,000 pounds. Obviously if you were an elephant hoping to shed a few pounds it would be worth taking the long trek from Angola to New Delhi. You'd sweat the pounds off on the grueling trip over in any case. Elephants are delicate creatures that walk almost noiselessly, with a smooth, rhythmic stride that absorbs their weight.

Slightly clumsier and with a wobbly gait, is third on the list of heavyweights, the white rhino. Take it from personal experience, if you see one coming don't stop to check out its color or temperament. Just run, preferably in zigzags, and live to see another day! Coming in next on the heavy list is the hippo, considered the most aggressive animal in Africa. Now here are more fascinating facts to help you deal with your weight issues. An adult male hippo weighs between 3,000 to 3,900 pounds while a more demure female tips the scale at 600 pounds less.

Hippos spend most of the day in the water, often asleep, and come out at night to graze. A hippo's diet consists almost entirely of grass and they usually graze for four to five hours each night, consuming on average about 90 pounds of grass. Still grass is grass. Not a helluva of lot of calories in it nor is it very appetizing. Now here's the really interesting part. A male hippo continues to put on weight throughout his life and the female peaks at twenty five. An old geezer hippo can rattle the scales at 7,000 pounds and sometimes breaks it at an incredible weight of 7,900 pounds.

He has more than doubled his weight. Why? He hasn't changed his diet, he's still eating the *same* amount of grass. No more and no less. He hasn't ducked out to rampage the local McDonalds so where did he go wrong? Nowhere. Nature just intended for him to get bigger as he aged, just as we do. What's more, a hippo has short stubby legs to carry his weight. Still, hippos don't need knee or hip replacements and at their best speed of 30mph they can outrun an Olympic sprinter.

To add a spanner in the works, the giraffe comes in at number five on the list of heavyweights. However the giraffe gets away with it because of his height. He's up rather than down, so he's the model of the animal kingdom and has rather an aloof air to go along with his rarefied sense of self. With that elongated neck he's bound to have his head in the clouds. Still you don't see the other animal species hanging around him longingly, hoping to morph into his slim leggyness.

Still we can learn from the example of the giraffe. May I suggest that next time you go to your doctor's office for a weigh in that you invest in a pair of stilts so that your weight will equal your height. These are the tricks of the trade. During my time in Nepal I never once spotted a giraffe because I was on the wrong continent however I did have my share of wonderful experiences. At the time of the Diwali festival, several rangers asked if I would become their adopted 'sister' as a mark of our bond. It was a true honor and of course I agreed.

As I was the only woman on the campsite, I offered to become sister to any of the men who wished it on the day. To my surprise all the men agreed and I ended up with sixty brothers! Then came another blessing. Aware of my love for Ana, her driver asked me to carry out the ceremony for the elephant. At his command she leant down, and waited patiently while I drew a red tikkha on her forehead. Not only did I end up with sixty brothers, I also have an elephant as a sister!

So there is no doubt as to my sacred animal totem, the one that inspires, guides and protects me. I am proud to be one of the elephant clan. I share their sensitivity, joy for life and above all, thick stubby knees. I can also charge like a crazed bull elephant if someone crosses me. Many tribal cultures, including the North American Indians and Australian Aborigines, are closely connected to nature and understand the importance of their animal guides. These empower them on life's journey and a person is often named after their totem to draw on their wisdom and strength, like Running Bear, White Eagle and Great Elk.

Even though we in Western society often distance ourselves from nature, we can still be in touch with our animal guides. When I was young mine was a deer. I had a little porcelain statue of one I had been given and which I treasured and kept near my bed. I loved to walk barefoot like a deer and feel the earth beneath my feet. I trod gently, not wanting to leave my footprints on the earth or make a sound.

As we progress in life our totems change because we need new lessons to grow and different sources to inspire us and provide us with strength. As I grew older I went from gentle deer to majestic eagle. I wanted to fly into the wind and explore every far region of the globe. To perch on a craggy rock and lead a wild solitary existence.

In the masterful book, 'The Clan of the Cave Bear' by Jean Auel, the heroine Ayla is cast out of her homeland by a natural disaster. All alone and desperate she goes in search of a place to belong. In a curious twist on the usual story, her tall slim Arian body,

11

blond hair and blue eyes are out of place when she chances upon the Cave Bear tribe from the south. The short dark tribe see her as downright ugly and weird.

It's all a question of perspective and what rocks in one place fails to deliver in another. One day Ayla strays onto cave lion territory. She is stalked by a lion and falls down a rock ledge in fright. Taking refuge in a small cave, she scrunches into a tight ball but the lion is no fool. He smells fresh meat so he stretches his large paw inside the rock opening and sinks his claws into her left thigh … four parallel deep gashes.

The tribe's magician Mog-ur is in a quandary when it comes time to choose the girl's animal totem. Ayla has obviously been touched by the spirit of the cave lion but how can he give the girl such a powerful totem? No man would be strong enough to handle it so the girl would never be able to find a mate. Despite the tribe's objections, the magician gives the girl the spirit of Ursus, the cave lion. He reasons that the animal has chosen her and besides the girl is so unattractive she will have no partner to protect her anyway. She *needs* to be strong.

So ladies choose your animal totem carefully because there will be lifelong repercussions. If you want to keep men away then I recommend selecting a snarling black jaguar or a stuffed wombat as your totem. Choosing a sloth or a tarantula might also do the trick. Men, think twice. The totem of a scared rabbit or a horny hare might just scare the ladies off. A stud bull could be equally daunting, or not.

Animals serve to remind us that we are each created differently. We come in assorted packages, with our own distinct temperament and mentality. We each thrive under different circumstances. Some like it hot while others revel in the cold. Some love the lay of the land, others frolic beneath the sea. That's what makes our world so wondrous.

Animals also remind us that we are exactly as we were created and no amount of huffing or puffing is going to alter your species. All you will succeed in doing in blowing hard is bringing your house down and yourself right along with it. No matter how much you try, you can never become what you were never meant to be. Rather you should be content as you are. This is the reality. Brand it into your consciousness.

IF YOU STARVE AN ELEPHANT IT WILL NEVER BECOME A GAZELLE. INSTEAD YOU WILL END UP WITH A WRINKLED OLD BAG. A VERY UNHAPPY, VEXED WRINKLED OLD BAG INSTEAD OF THE GRAND REGAL ELEPHANT IT WAS BORN TO BE. YOU CANNOT CHANGE OR MORPH SPECIES. *NOR SHOULD YOU ASPIRE TO.*

That poor starved elephant will be forced to resort to expensive and extensive surgery to get rid of the folds of saggy skin left behind after its unhappy ordeal. It's not natural or healthy to go to extremes but it's wonderful to be *your* optimum self, to revel in your own body shape and to hone it to perfection. Watch your frustration melt right along with all the excess baggage. Yes, it's wonderful to be yourself.

Man appears to be the only creature that is so discontent with his own body that he attempts to transform it into an alien form and distort his original self image. This self deprecation is not inherent in his nature but rather is a learned response. Where does this lack of confidence and personal disdain come from? The title of this woman's magazine article will give you a clue. 'Learn to love the body bits you hate.' This sort of hype contributes to the erosion of our self esteem.

Animals are not so insecure. That's not to say they don't like to look their personal best. Most enjoy preening to make the most of their looks or to attract a partner. Just look at the magnificent display of the lyre bird. The male spreads his stunning turquoise tail to attract a mate, capitalizing on his inherited good looks. He does not resort to sticking himself with a twig to inject toxin into his body or plucking his feathers to alter his appearance. Rather he relies on the beauty nature gave him.

He recognizes his own magnificence while we have trouble seeing our own. Does a lion roll over in a field of poppies after a downpour to change his mane from golden to red? NO, he prefers to lie down in a patch of sunflowers that reflects his own radiance. Does a chimp look into a mirror and screech in horror? Does he rush off to the salon for waxing to remove unwanted hair or to the dentist to have his teeth straightened? No, rather he falls in love with his own reflection.

We humans are rarely content. The lighter of our lot bask in the sun to tan a golden brown or spray paint their body in varying shades of caramel or mocha, a sign of beauty and a decadent lifestyle. Meanwhile darker races rush out to buy skin whiteners to erase their heritage and become silky white which in their cultures denotes a rich lifestyle. Affluent people starve themselves to look thin while the leaner races fatten themselves up as a sign of a beauty and wealth.

Consider this interesting fact. A bear hibernates in a cave for several months of the year. It has no food or water. Does it emerge after its time at the mountain spa, trim, taught and terrific, happy with its new found self? Even though it might be several pounds lighter it prefers it's old self and will soon return to its NORMAL bulky weight after it guzzles itself silly as a result of being deprived of sustenance for so long. The bear is a good example of the ultimate yoyo dieter.

Which leads us to the subject of exercise. We were not all born to bolt through the bushes like an overexcited wart hog or a speedy cheetah hunting down a wildebeest. Have you ever watched a koala on any given day? It barely blinks, let alone moves. I thought the docile little creature was perpetually spaced out on gum leaves but after a visit to a wildlife park in the Australian bush, the ranger informed me that their diet affords them little energy and they can hardly make the effort.

We have much to learn from animals. Some species hunt in packs like wolves, move in herds like cattle or sheep or swim in pods like dolphins. Most birds fly in a flock while ants and bees prefer colonies. Others animals live solitary lives, content to be on their own. Tigers rule over a large territory to prowl in and will tolerate no intruders in their space. Like the legendary Greta Garbo, they want to be alone.

While we cherish the variety in animals we are unable to accept the diversity in our own kind and to treasure it. It's the ultimate HIPPO-CRACY. Man will fight to the death to save the whales but then want to shoot down any person carrying too much blubber!

Nonsense. They are valued members of society and deserve much greater respect.

Furthermore we are not all sprinters nor do we all aspire to climb mountains or jump out of moving aircraft. We are not all addicted to treadmills, pounding a million miles on the endless road to nowhere. The only animals foolish enough to do so are hamsters and rats because they're frightfully bored and have nowhere else to go. Or else they're deranged because they've been locked up for so long. No other animals would waste their time. With no other motivation than to go round and round in circles most would prefer to go hang out on a rock or on a cliff face and swoop down on their prey only when they need a good feed.

Animals rarely exercise just for the heck of it or because they have to. Rather they move with purpose, out of necessity and out of joy. Elephants dance, swans glide, antelopes cavort, monkeys play, fish swish, eagles soar, bulls charge, horses bolt, rabbits and deer frolic, badger's burrow, beavers build, birds fly, bees buzz and butterflies flutter. We all do it differently in our own sublime magnificent way. The trick is writing your own music and discovering the tune.

A ROCKY ROAD

Acceptance of self is hard, especially when it has been whipped out of you at an early age. Why Western society is so self defeating remains a mystery. When one half of the population is treated with contempt by the other half, who according to our version of reality has copped the good end of the stick from the start, it is a travesty.

I grew up in the sixties, an exciting time when much of the world was covered with a mantle of love and freedom and the rest was being torn apart. It was an age of exploration, pushing the boundaries and of self discovery. I was lost in the music and the wonder of it all. If only I could transcend into the ethereal Stevie Nicks of Fleetwood Mac or willowy Michelle Phillips and glide across the stage. And the universe.

Instead I was grateful for the bulk of Mama Cass who was a true inspiration with her chunky size, flowing caftans and mellow voice. Until she supposedly choked on a ham sandwich and died. Like Elvis she loved her food. It was a healthier way to go considering most singers at the time succumbed to a lethal cocktail of sex, drugs and alcohol. In the midst of the decade came the onslaught of the perky slim blonds. It started off with the likes of Sandra Dee, Gidget, surfer movies and wholesome sun bleached teens. When Little Pattie sang, 'He's my blond headed, real gone surfer boy,' I cringed. I was a short, chubby Mediterranean and they were few and far between.

Granted there was busty Annette Funicello on the Mickey Mouse Club and the crooner Frankie Avalon, but the more mature Italian beauties like Gina Lollobrigida and Sophia Loren were sultry vixens who were way out of my reach. With breasts like ripe watermelons, killer lips and waists the size of a bottle top, I could scarcely relate.

So I was forced to alter my looks to fit in and learn to sew so that I had something groovy to wear. When I headed off to Manly beach with my friends, I hid behind dark sunglasses and a long blond wig. Unable to see, I hacked the front into a fringe. With the first breeze it stood up at attention but I didn't care because I fitted in with the rest.

Then I met Boris, a six foot tall beatnik with black beard, grey cashmere sweater and subtle intellect. I lost the wig and reverted to being dark and intense. As we strolled along the street hand in hand, I felt really cool. I could finally be myself and it was my mind that Boris found most attractive. However being deep and meaningful was not enough to sustain a teenage girl, especially in such an exciting era.

With the emergence of Twiggy in the 60's, the bug eyed blonde model with the body of a waif, most of the population was doomed. How could I ever be like her? By this time I was besotted with the Beatles and being chubby I could never compete with millions of other girls for their affection. Maybe they were evolved enough to recognize my inner beauty even if it was stuffed into a tight paisley mini dress.

Each Saturday my best friend Gisele and I would go to Channel Nine television studios to dance to the latest pop hits. As the camera added a few pounds, it was best not to watch yourself on the monitor. As aspiring groupies we scaled fire escapes and haunted hotel lobbies to get close to the stars. When an entire hotel floor was closed off for the Rolling Stones, Gisele, a nimble Gemini, furled herself up into a pretzel position and stowed away in the dumb waiter winching her way up to the barred floor. I, being a well endowed Libra, couldn't fit.

So began a long and tortuous relationship with my weight. Born under the sign of the scales, they were to rule my life for a very long time. So were mirrors, which I avoided, calorie counters, apple cider vinegar, grapefruit and even a brief stint with laxatives and diet pills. Libra is the symbol of balance so it was a question of finding the right one. Not so much for me but rather for society. With a large chunk of the population invalidated the scales were stacked against reason.

Trendy shops like Cue and John and Merivale stocked their dazzling designs up to a lean size 8. They were definitely not designed for plump girls or the average ones either. Forced to starve myself to shimmy into a fabulous purple satin or ruffled canary yellow mini dress, I tortured myself daily by peering into the scale's deep abyss willing the pounds to drop off. Instead I ended up peering into the deep abyss of my soul wondering why society rejected and wanted to punish me.

A nagging question dawned on me at the time, one that has hounded me ever since. Why did I have to starve myself to the point of extinction while all the designers had to do was to cut a piece of fabric bigger? It seemed by far the easier option. Luckily I was strong enough to carve out my own path in life but the rejection still hurt.

Sensibly I went to university and graduated at twenty. I majored in Psychology to understand the meaning of life and History to try and figure out how we had got it so wrong. It was not a time of romance but rather study because my looks had still not come into vogue. I was forever plagued by the feeling that I didn't belong in my society. A few years later it all fell into place when I discovered a love for Astrology which I went on to study in depth. Suddenly everything started to make sense and there was order in disorder and a meaning to life.

It helped me overcome all the challenges I had to face over the years and to discover a sense of self. I was fortunate to be bolstered by a strong ego and a belief in a higher power. I was also lucky that during my formative years at school that I was never singled out, harassed or teased in any way. It helped that I went to an all girl school and that my classmates were not the nasty type. Most came from various cultural backgrounds and were each individual in their own way.

The only thorn in my side at school was the gym class. Self conscious, I refused to get undressed in front of the other girls or wear a swimming costume. My breasts were by this time buoyant and my upper arms looked like they had floaties attached to them even though they didn't. To compound the problem was my ineptitude and dislike for sports and gymnastics. I found the whole idea of exerting myself in such a horrid way unnatural and abandoned the very thought.

It was as if I had been a pampered princess in a previous lifetime and now I was required to swing a bat. That was for heathens and gladiators. As for scaling and climbing, I believed the only thing worth mounting was a bed. Why run or sprint when you would work up a sweat and smell? And where exactly were you going? Why race when a leisurely stroll would get you to the same place, much more refreshed and ready for afternoon tea? It's a delicate Libran thing.

Still there was more to it. As a child I spent hours trying to master a forward roll. I thought about it a lot but couldn't quite wrap my mind around doing a pretzel roll with my body. It seemed such an unnatural ambition so in the end I gave up. I was completely incapable of it and found the whole idea rather bizarre. At school I forged notes to avoid gym class. I couldn't jump over wooden horses and always missed the softball when I tried to hit it, much to everyone's amusement.

The gym teacher ridiculed me mercilessly but I compensated with thoughts that creative and intellectual types are rarely athletic. It took many years for me to discover that I was born with a dodgy cerebellum at the base of my brain which accounted for my distorted balance and coordination since birth. It's impossible to uncover all the secrets of the universe or understand all the wounds we carry that make us distinct individuals. Instead we must honor our life journey, such as it is.

Others with more fragile egos did not fare so well when growing up. A friend's account of her childhood showed just how hurt and damaged she'd been by destructive others. Debra came from a 'large' family and even though she ate no more than other girls she was bigger than the rest. At school she was left on her own, with few friends. So in order to survive she withdrew into a private place where she was safe.

Her sense of alienation grew with the cruel jibes of the gym teacher. I could relate to her story as she spoke because I too was made fun of by mine. To compound the situation, children born under the fuller signs of the zodiac are often the artistic, intellectual or musical types and are usually not athletic. To be forced to do something as foreign as gymnastics is as embarrassing as it can be excruciating.

Debra was devastated when her gym teacher called her names in front of the whole class and mockingly compared her to her older sister who shared her aversion to sports. Publicly and constantly humiliated, Debra retreated further into her shell. She was not equipped to deal with a society that had no place for her nor did she want to in the end.

As a sensitive Pisces Debra had a wonderful imagination and drew on it in order to cope. As she grew older Debra was able to better recognize her beauty even though her ego had been worn down over the years. She found solace in music and was a gifted singer although she still grappled with issues of self esteem throughout her life.

Bigger children often take a terrible blow to their ego growing up. From an early age they feel different and lacking and are sensitized to the fact by the attitude of others. One lovely young Leo endured endless bullying at school because of her size. It peaked when a picture of a whale was posted on a notice board with her name splashed across it. This was the work of a malicious fool, desperate for attention and in need of a misguided ego boost at the expense of another.

Bullying knows no boundaries. In the hands of the insecure and aggressive it is brutal and unkind. It's not restricted to the overweight or the slight but rather singles out its victims at random. It is aimed at those who are perceived to be weak or vulnerable, or different or better in some way. It preys on the sensitive and the more highly evolved soul who present a threat to those less worthy or those who are truly weak.

It's cold comfort but with a shift of perspective, your thinking can be reprogrammed to see beyond the cruel words and put downs. To be called a whale is obviously intended to be insulting but in truth the opposite is true because whales are highly valued creatures. People fight hard to preserve them and pay to go out in boats to watch them frolic in the ocean, while undersized fish are thrown back overboard till they thrive and nasty predatory sharks are hunted down and slain.

Yes, it's all about perspective. Never allow anyone to hurt you, defame, denounce or shame you in any way. If anyone needs to be ashamed it's these folk and their words and actions will come back to haunt them one day. My advice to those wounded souls who came to me for counseling was to imagine the hostile person holding up a mirror and looking at themselves, for in truth their words were a reflection of their own inner being and their damaged state of mind.

Abuse takes many forms and is more lethal when it comes from someone we care for and respect. This is all the worse when the hurt and disapproval comes from a family member, especially a parent. If that parent is an Aries or Capricorn they often can't help themselves.

The tougher signs of the ram and goat are naturally thin and even more naturally critical. They want everyone to be lean like themselves and they have no qualms about letting you know it, over and over again. Oh pity the gentle child who lives under a ram gone wild or a stuffy old goat. Often they can eat whatever they want and graze all day unlike their fuller offspring who may eat very little but pay the price.

One larger lady I spoke to, elegant and attractive in her own right, had a hellish childhood growing up with an Aries mother. Ironically she was a Capricorn herself, an exception to the thin rule because many of her planets were situated in the more ample signs. Capricorn and Aries square each other in a horoscope, forming a difficult ninety degree angle between them, so there was a natural tension between mother and daughter which manifested mostly around mealtimes.

The only plump child among thin siblings she was deprived and made to go without by her mother so she could look like the rest of the family, forced to conform to become slim and acceptable. No butter on her sandwiches, no cookies or cakes when the rest were tucking into them and at the family barbecue, a nice piece of grilled fish instead of sizzling sausages or a juicy steak. She was definitely made to feel different, not in a good way and so her inferiority complex began.

Despite her father's protest that she should be treated like the rest, her Aries mum was having none of it. She wasn't going to be seen with a tubby child, ashamed or what might be seen as a poor reflection of herself. It's a curious thing that in the animal kingdom it's the runt of the litter, the scrawny one that gets neglected and often left to die. It seems that some people turn their back on the healthiest of the brood, the chubby, robust one. The reverse is true in some poorer cultures where family fatten their children as a sign of affluence and health.

The sharp words of a critical parent often hound you into a sad adulthood, leaving an indelible painful groove in your psyche. Such a deep hurt can never truly go away. It may be a subtle yet traumatic blow to the ego. 'You've put on a bit of weight lately,' dad says as you reach across for the potatoes at the dinner table. 'Do you really need that cookie?' mum asks casually as she munches on a carrot stick. It passes down through the generations, comments aimed at a plump grandchild through you of course. And so the myth perpetuates. As does the hurt.

Then society gets in on the act or more accurately it may have contrived it in the first place. With an emphasis on outer appearance those who don't conform to society's expectations bear the brunt and may be bullied and called derisive names. Like any misfit, anyone who doesn't conform to the mould of the time, they suffer. Nerds retreat into books or cyber space for comfort. The deeper types may become Goths and withdraw into a dark place that reflects the confusion and turmoil in their soul. The rebellious sort will do their own thing and thumb their nose at society, and hopefully not become serial killers as the anger inside them explodes in a torrent of misguided rage.

A child is astute enough to know when they don't fit in, especially when they are forced to face adult issues before their time. Girls know when they don't look like Sleeping Beauty, the demure blonde princess. Some boys are so damaged they believe they resemble the beast rather than the prince in fairy tales. These children's self image becomes warped because of these impossible stereotypes.

In high school I loved to act and drama class was my favorite. I wanted to play Titania, the queen of the fairies in Midsummer Night's Dream but I didn't have the ethereal looks. Instead I was cast as the dim witted male Bottom, sorely denting my ego. It was a far meatier role but at that stage I needed to have my beauty acknowledged.

Teenage movies which feature the ugly duckling or outcast usually have only two possible outcomes. One, a group of bitchy prom queens will come down from their ivory tower long enough to deign to rescue the poor unfortunate lass. She will be transformed from her plain drab self into her fabulous alter ego. She will knock everyone's socks off as she struts through the school corridors, with her hair bouffed up, all dressed to kill and her lips coated in lip gloss, singing happy tunes.

Just as the ugly duckling turned into a swan, and Cinderella was lifted from her dreary life sweeping up ashes to marry a prince, she is resurrected. The next scenario comes from the mind of a Scorpio director. In the darker version, the much maligned misfit is so filled with rage she goes on the rampage. From a page out of a Stephen King novel she will burn the school down with one volatile glare or the wave of her hand and annihilate all those who have ever victimized her. Her nails will either be painted blood red or ebony black.

Now look at the real situation. The rejected person will retreat within their own soul, hurt and struggling to find a true sense of self. They search for a shred of hope which may come through a kind-hearted teacher, a positive parent or supportive friends. Hopefully their ego is strong enough to recognize its own beauty and uniqueness. Talents will overflow and the soul will grow and bask in the aura of its own greatness. This is the best case scenario.

During my work as a teacher and school counselor that was rarely the case. The children referred to me came for many different reasons but they were all damaged in their own way or had simply lost their way. Never was size the determining factor because emotional problems manifest in a multitude of behaviors, do not conform to a certain shape or size and are mirrored in a whole range of human conditions.

When an ego is battered because of the way a person looks, it is a senseless waste because it has been cast down by society's hand. Confronted by unrealistic role models, who by their very nature make us feel less than we are, it is difficult to stay on top. Only the hardiest ego will endure the onslaught to thrive and to live an authentic life.

There is a positive edge to the journey of the outcast. Through suffering and introspection they develop depth and understanding of the human condition. They feel pain therefore they develop compassion, they are hurt and so they reach out to others in need. Hopefully they learn to recognize that real beauty lies within and radiates on the outside. Beauty arises from a genuine state of being and living in truth.

Those who sail through life without challenge often turn out to be vacant and shallow, concentrating on the materialistic aspects of life. Some of today's so-called 'celebrities' possess all the depth of a thimble. Why on earth would we aspire to be like them when most of us already possess far more substance than they will ever know? They have had it far too easy and few have suffered except for the misery they have cast down upon themselves. The true icons of our times, like Marilyn Monroe, James Dean and Michael Jackson, self destructed from the pressure. They were beautiful but tortured souls. They teach us to be at peace with ourselves.

THE TRUTH IS NO MATTER HOW OTHERS PERCEIVE YOU IT'S ONLY IMPORTANT HOW YOU SEE YOURSELF.

FAT IS A
THREE LETTER WORD

Fat is treated in our society like an aberration, to be avoided like a deadly plague. Traditionally the only big people considered acceptable were, and still are to some degree, comedians or singers. Stout male comedians of our time include the classic W.C. Fields, Oliver Hardy, Fatty Arbuckle, Jackie Gleason, Benny Hill, Dom deLuise, Divine, Drew Carey, Jack Black, John Belushi and John Goodman.

Comely ladies that made us laugh include Mae West, Dawn French, the Two Fat Ladies, Jo Brand, Jennifer Saunders, Dame Edna Everage, Roseanne Barr and Rosie O'Donnell and a batch of others. They each have a rather caustic edge to them, and you'd be bitter too if you were treated by society in such a disdainful way.

Most of us can identify with their angst. The cheeky Aussie star Magda Szubanski who was on TV in Big Ladies Blouse and then the popular series Kath and Kim, also played the portly farmer's wife in Babe and the voice of a penguin in Happy Feet. Despite her larger size, she was voted Australia's most popular television personality.

Other large people are saved by their voice. Society begrudgingly accepts that big chested people house a powerful instrument. Mama Cass crooned, Aretha Franklin belts out gutsy R and B demanding Respect, Luciano Pavarotti and Joan Sutherland sang with voices that transported us to a higher realm, Jennifer Hudson and Jordan Sparks wowed us with their tremendous talent while Meatloaf roared like a Bat out of Hell. Big is powerful, with a message to boot.

Singers are governed by the sign of Taurus which rules the throat. Its symbol, the bull, is fierce with a wonderful proud chest. Many singers are large passionate people, be they stars, back-up singers or members of a gospel choir. Opera singers are larger than life and as we know, 'it's not over till the fat lady sings.' Even if she can't fit into Carmen's dress and has to endure the barbs of a critical producer.

More and more opera singers have been ostracized for their size and are not deemed suitable for certain roles, despite their magnificent voices. Their weight is blamed on erratic work hours, excessive travel and comfort eating. Not true. The astrology chart I cast for an opera singer at the Sydney Opera House was a typical example, revealing that the planet Venus was conjunct Pluto in her horoscope.

Basically this means that the feminine energy of Venus was joined with the masterful energy of Pluto at the time of her birth. As one astrology text states, 'this strong Venus placement brings artistic talent, expressed through combined drama-music, such as opera.' As a serious musical form, opera demands a powerful presence. Pluto bestows a charismatic glow that radiates throughout the theatre.

Opera singers are not meant to shrink on stage. Imagine if Pavarotti was reed thin? His presence was magnetic and his voice flooded the theatre to fill the hearts and minds of people. When the acclaimed Greek soprano Maria Callas drastically shed over sixty pounds in 1954, her voice suffered irreparably and her career was cut short. Her voice shrunk along with her body and her vanity proved her undoing.

With articles like this one that appeared in the Arts Section of the UK Guardian newspaper, it's surprising that we're not all consumed with rightful indignation. When people are belittled because of their size and their talent overlooked it is not only despicable it is a mockery. However the shame belongs to the writer and not to his target.

'Why the fat lady can't sing,' the writer begins. 'Perhaps the decision by the Royal Opera House to sack a soprano for being too fat should be seen as a heroic action in the worldwide war on obesity. Opera singers are practically the only people in the world, together with darts players and sumo wrestlers, who actually rejoice in their fatness.

'American research shows that obesity causes 400,000 deaths in the US each year. Far more deaths than the terrorists of the world could ever hope to achieve. (What an appalling statement!) The only way of attacking this problem is to instill shame and fear into those who eat too much but opera singers seem to be immune to these emotions.'

Is this pathetic writer for real? I have visions of him nibbling on a cream cracker and blue vein cheese while spilling a glass of red wine over his computer. Personally I'd like to tie him to his chair and force feed him a truckload of pork pies with lashings of cheesecake to follow. How sanctimonious and how condescending! This is terrorism at its worst. The kind that shoots you down in flames and destroys your soul. We wonder why larger people have complexes and low self esteem. Now we begin to understand why they have to laugh so as not to cry and why they sing loudly so they can reconnect to the higher power that created them. One who rejoices in His creation and His image.

A perfect example of the ego being worn down is Paul Potts who appeared on the UK show 'Britain's Got Talent.' A quiet, unassuming Libran he worked selling mobile phones. His looks did not inspire him with confidence yet when he opened his mouth he was transformed. As were we all. His superb operatic voice flooded the studio with light and the audience was transfixed. His is a remarkable talent.

When his first album One Chance was released it skyrocketed to number one in the album charts, outselling the rest of the top ten combined. It was not only his voice that attributed to his success but also the fact that he was a normal man, a humble person with an exceptional gift. He had been bullied at school because of his looks and was so beaten down he tossed a coin to see if he should compete. Paul's horoscope shows the same aspect as my opera singer friend. However in his chart, Pluto joins with the masculine Mars to endow him with that special presence needed to enchant audiences.

More recently on the same English show, matronly Susan Boyle left her mark when she sang the very apt song, 'I dreamed a dream'. Her stunning voice distinguished her but even more remarkable was her humble persona and wit. Susan is a reminder that the extraordinary can lay hidden, waiting to emerge like a dazzling butterfly from its cocoon. So the audience took to her, hoping that one day they too could shine. Then the pressure of instant success and adulation got too much for her, along with the need to make her over to create a marketable asset, and so she cracked. To go from being overlooked most of your life to the fickle pleasures of the limelight is daunting at best.

When it comes to society's obsession with a person's looks, what I fail to understand is why the two extremes of body shape get the most coverage, like two polar opposites with nothing in between. Like Laurel and Hardy and Abbot and Costello, there appears to be only fat and thin. They make up a perfect 10 but the trouble is the thin people are 'number one' and large ones are a 'big fat zero'.

And that sums it up. But what about all those people who lie in between. Most of the population in fact. Why are this silent majority misrepresented in the media, if featured at all? Where are the normal inbetweeners? Why are our screens and magazines not flooded with healthy role models of vivacious happy people of an average size?

And WHO exactly dictates what we are meant to look like? I have no idea who this silent manipulator is, yanking at our strings as if we are helpless puppets. It's as if an alien race zoomed down to earth one cloudy night and embedded our brains with strange imperfect images that hardly resemble humans. At least most I know.

Look at the pale skeletal models who strut down our runways scowling, as if they're suffering from a case of massive moral reflux after being starved of any real sustenance, body or soul. Their sullen looks reflect their disillusionment and the catastrophe that fashion has become. Bearing little resemblance to the average person, we may as well be looking at that alien race for all the relevance they have.

At the last fashion show I chanced upon at the shopping mall, I was more captivated by the sea of faces in the audience rather than the catatonic stance of the models. Staring mindlessly at the lanky tall women who strutted their stuff were a disenchanted bunch of chubby short folk, pregnant women and an assorted throng of people who regretted their recent binge in the food court. The clothes were not designed for real people nor were we designed for them. Instead of elevating us, these fashions diminish us.

It's time for a long overdue reality check. No longer do we crave perfect images of the young miss or sexy diva who plays the heroine alongside the handsome lead in a romantic comedy. Interestingly less attractive men get away with being cast in the lead when they play on their imperfections or quirkiness but women less than perfect are rarely tolerated. It's an unacceptable double standard that indicates that men are considered to have appealing qualities like humor or character whereas women are judged almost solely on their looks.

Then there are those distorted images of overweight people who cake themselves with slapstick and self mockery, in those films that present fat people as moronic caricatures. They pad their stars out in synthetic fat suits to ridicule them even more. They are the butt of every joke and every derisive comment, which they apparently deserve when they are coated in gel and pumped up to look like a bloated fish.

Movies like Big Fat Momma, Norbit, the Nutty Professor and Shallow Hal reflect society's abhorrence of fat. How disgusting to see Gwyneth Paltrow thunder about on wobbly synthetic thighs like a mass of heaving jello. The writers missed the point. It was not that Hal could not recognize the beauty within but rather they who slaughtered it. In doing so they offended any theatre goer with an ounce of fat or sensitivity and reduced the subject of weight to a whole new base level.

The show Hairspray shows a bouncy plus size lass who is so bubbly she appears to have drunk a few too many bottles of happy juice or has ducked out behind the kitchen to sniff the cellulite cream. She is so upbeat she hasn't realized she's different to the rest. To her credit she just doesn't care. She sees herself as beautiful so expects everyone else to. As for John Travolta puffed up in layers of gunk to play mum, all that goo impinged on his vocal chords sending him from baritone to soprano. Get a real big fat momma to play mum and watch us smile.

Film is catching up with popular opinion at a very grinding pace. Films like Real Women Have Curves with the lovely America Ferrara are welcome. Unfortunately Hollywood took a Latin soap opera star and transformed her into Ugly Betty. Looking purposely dowdy, America is only a mere size six. Sara Paul was a stunning redhead with a hint of curves in the TV series Less than Perfect. A beautiful size eight (less than the US average) Sara was bullied by the media and referred to as overweight. She succumbed to pressure, shrunk in size and dyed her hair. She then fizzled into the background as just another Hollywood blonde. Hopefully she'll revert back to type soon.

Another Sara who did not fare well was Sarah Ferguson, once married to Prince Andrew, the Duke of York. Cruelly dubbed 'the Duchess of Pork', Fergie was another Libran, a naturally curvy sign. Personally I find her angular shape less pleasing but she is under more pressure than most to conform. It was reported that Fergie feared that her daughter Beatrice would become anorexic after cruel remarks in the press about her figure, even though she is a healthy size 10.

Gradually larger people are being slipped into a number of TV programs, usually in the background. The bulkier secretary in an ill fitting suit, the surly lawyer or the bubbly side kick who provides a little humor or angst. Isn't it about time that the sexy star is average or plus size, like lovely Kathy Bates who candidly displayed her naked body to Jack Nicholson in the hot tub, in the film About Schmidt. Let's see a *real* woman brimming with life who captures the heart of a *real* man who appreciates her essential beauty. Or a woman who creates magic in her life, whatever that may be or she chooses it to be.

Fat on screen usually represents someone who is slovenly or who possesses a mean temper or sarcastic humor. A good example was the show Roseanne, where the star Roseanne Barr paraded her sloppy demeanor, sharp tongue and acid wit for the world to see. Jackie Gleason was mean tempered and loud mouthed in the Honeymooners, while the chubby Edina in the British show Absolutely Fabulous was a total lush giving way to her baser appetites and showing no self control in her quest for gratification. Her gaunt sidekick Patsy doesn't fare much better but then again she didn't eat. Her preferred diet was cigarettes and booze, anything to stay lean and caustic.

The Australian hit show Kath and Kim was based on a dysfunctional mother and daughter. Kath the mother was thin, bubbly and energetic, while floozy daughter Kim with her bulging tummy and exposed g-string was always foraging in the cupboard for anything she could stuff her face with. In the US version, Kath retained her brisk leanness but Kim didn't fare so well. Casting Selma Blair as Kim and asking her to pack on a few pounds for the role meant she looked even lovelier, so the show lost its oomph. If Selma Blair's slim body is the result of hours of binge eating let us all head off to the cupboard!

Show us a naturally rounded beauty like the delectable Jennifer Coolidge, best known for playing Stifler's mum in the hit movie American Pie and the zany manicurist in Legally Blond. She is a beautiful woman with a delightful sense of humor. Though she often plays ditzy roles, she does them with panache and looks just fabulous.

When fat suits are used in movies to portray real people it insults our intelligence. In reality the only ones who are pumped up are thin folk. They insert silicone breasts to look more like the goddess Venus who did not endow them with curves at birth. As they age their fine skin, not bolstered by sumptuous fat cells, starts to sag until it collapses. Then it is pumped up with collagen and fillers. Lips, butts, brows, breasts. Every body part has to be primed to regain its lost youth.

Big people finally get their day. They age better because their fat cells provide a buffer. Despite reaching my golden age, I have very few wrinkles. I am still called miss and have been mistaken for being much younger. My partner of ten years was a gorgeous man twenty years my junior. His girlfriend prior to me was a top model but he had no issues with my weight. He reminded me every day just how beautiful I was and stated wisely that one recognizes the beauty in the one they love.

When people are portrayed as fat and blowsy, and unsightly photos taken to prove the point, there is a collective grimace. And just the slightest hint of voyeurism in case, heaven forbid, we might turn out that way one day. We sigh at images of Kirstie Alley as she descends into 'fat hell.' She has let herself go or so the candid photos of her devouring a hamburger or donut suggest. Then again photos of spindly young starlets looking like they've just crawled out of a garbage bin or groveling in the gutter after a drunken night out, do us no favors.

I recently watched a HBO movie aptly titled To Be Fat Like Me. Picture this alarming scenario. Blond, athletic daughter and potential prom queen detests her mother because she was once fat and ate cakes which ultimately led to a near fatal heart attack. She verbally abuses her mother to the point of denigration and promises never to become like her by drinking health shakes and running around in circles.

Poor mum is at her wit's end, although the young chubby brother fares better. Daughter reserves her hatred for mum for allowing her brother to have pizza nights and an extra slice of cake every now and then. Circumstances conspire to put daughter out of action, obviously the great Almighty's attempt to instill some humility in his young creation. So with nothing better to do, daughter embarks on a school project with a friend to see what it feels like to be fat.

She dons the regulation fat suit and plasters some concoction on her face to puff her up. On her sojourn as a fatty she is the butt of abuse and derision and soon despairs at the way it makes her feel and how shallow most of the population is. Funny I have been a size 16 most of my life and never experienced one nasty comment or sideway glance. Probably because I live in a society where my size is the norm, even though my society refuses to accept this openly or graciously.

In her quest for understanding, daughter befriends two outcasts. A male nerd and a plump lass who displays ten times the depth of emotion of her bony counterpart, having been forced to introspect most of her life about the anomalies of the human condition. Daughter rationalizes her ruse by saying, 'You can't fix what you don't understand.' Which begs the question of why she thinks she has the right to do so and does the issue need fixing or are larger people just meant to be that way?

Not only is the daughter sanctimonious but also the fundamental premise of the movie. The first shot shows mum cooking up a fat infested breakfast of melted butter, a batch of fried eggs and sizzling bacon and calorie laden hotcakes. Then some random shots of chubby brother stuffing his face with a whole pizza and her plump friend's stash of hidden chocolate bars in the glove box of her car.

Give me a break! Can you guarantee me that the scrawny family next door don't eat the same lardy breakfast or call in for greasy take away seven nights a week? And that thin people don't eat chocolate to keep them on a constant high! Don't be fooled for a moment. All the large people I know are careful about their diets, out of fear of retribution or packing on the pounds. The thinnest friend I have never stops stuffing junk food into her mouth barely stopping to take a breath.

This is the dangerous stereotypical thinking that has to be erased from society's consciousness. When shows like Two and a Half Men portray the son Jake as a human garbage bin, with a weight problem caused by his insatiable and voracious appetite, this misguided premise is reinforced. That fat is caused entirely by overeating and is the folly of a person who has no self control or dignity. Think again.

My sister grew up as a thin gangly child but as soon as she hit puberty, the hormones kicked in and she bloated in size. No amount of diets or food deprivation has made the slightest difference because food was not the deciding variable. To this day she eats sparingly but still has to deal with her share of cruel jibes, mostly from supercilious medics who insinuate her size is of her own making. Still with a strong Leo ascendant she has risen above it to finally accept who she is.

The film To Be Fat Like Me redeemed itself by ending with the profound line, 'The world will tell you who you are until *you* tell the world.' It's all about attitude. Refuse to buy into the hype that you have created your own misery by eating more than anyone else and therefore somehow deserve to suffer. You know deep down who you were meant to be so conduct yourself with integrity and pride.

One of Australia's top models in the sixties was the lovely Maggie Tabberer. Over the years her lean body shape blossomed into a larger size, a natural progression over time. She did not pout nor did she unravel. Instead she turned it around. A picture of elegance and decorum, Maggie is a sound role model for the larger sized woman.

She carved out a fashion empire based on plus sizes and headed a popular woman's magazine for some years. No one ever comments about her size or shape because she looks good and besides she simply would not stand for it. Instead they concentrate on her accomplishments and her considerable expertise. As they should.

Others have done the same. Delta Burke from the US program Designing Woman had a similar weight gain but still looked attractive, although she had issues accepting the shift at first. She ended up designing a stunning lingerie line for the fuller figure. It was a hard road for her when she gained weight and she nearly became unstuck but she turned it around to triumph in the end and made the most of it.

Donald Trump is rich enough not to care what anyone thinks about his hair and the confident ones get to call the shots. So believe in who you are and take a leaf out of Miss Piggy's book. Be fabulous. Don't let anyone or anything stand in your way. Fling your hair about in wild abandon and stomp on any little toads or insects that annoy you. Remember one thing. It's not only in the presentation but also what lies beneath. Good things like diamonds may come in small packages but always remember, the larger the carat the more valuable.

So sparkle, shimmer, gleam, radiate and shine. Yes, shine on.

THE O WORD

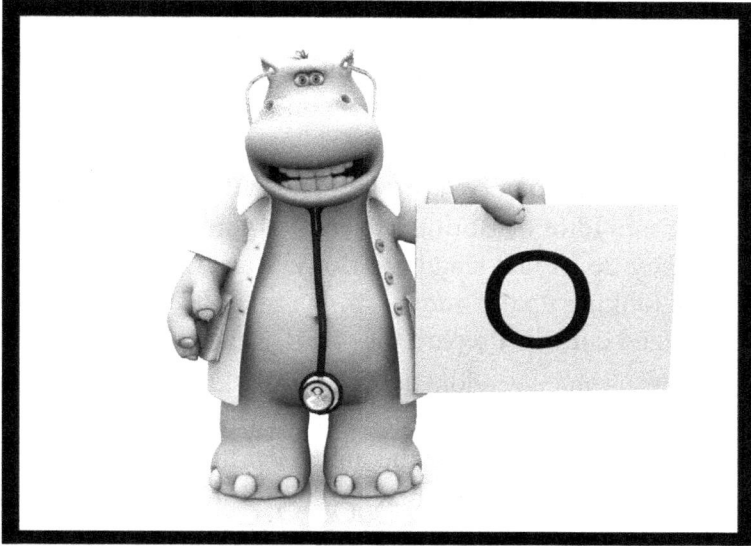

Here's something that can definitely snuff out your light. The dreaded O word. Hands up all those who have heard it. When you're standing in the doctor's office, baring your soul as well as your body, and he looks you up and down as if he's about to select a shank of meat for the weekend barbecue. Then baste you on the spit. His lips quiver and your body starts to shiver and then out pops the dreaded O word. OBESE.

You shrink into a tiny ball hoping that you can curl your fat cells up and tuck them away in the lining of your shoe. You blink three times desperate to dispel the image, hoping that you imagined the whole awful scene. The doctor nods his head again, confirming his original damning diagnosis. Yep. You've got it. You've got 'obese'. Your soul melts into mulch as your cellulite starts to self destruct. It's too late.

You've got 'obese'.

The doctor breaks the news to you as if he's the only person on the face of the planet to have ever seen you properly or you've been too scared to ever look into a mirror to see yourself. Exactly what has he based this spectacular diagnosis on? A cursory glance or did he take out his weapon of choice and measure your fat? Clutch a clump of it in his metal pincers while sighing out loud. His lips start to form a word.

Or at least three very nasty letters. BMI. They could stand for Brutal Moronic Idiot or Boring Miserable Ingrate for all the damage they do. They do in fact stand for Body Mass Index, which sounds like you're looking up the number for an undertaker who specializes in roomy sized coffins. Prepare for one if your BMI is high.

In all its ultimate wisdom the WHO (World Health Organization) introduced the BMI as the universal standard of weight. (As if there could be a single standard for the entire world with all its divergent shapes, sizes, genes and cultures). The BMI measures one's weight in pounds divided by the square of one's height in inches. Now I'm not good with figures on any given day, especially my own, but that's lousy. I don't want to be compared to a leggy Scandinavian lap dancer or a scant Thai one for that matter.

What about my breasts? They're inherited so they deserve special dispensation. On my travels around the world I met the rest of my clan and they were all blessed with one distinguishing feature. Killer breasts. Not ample breasts but gynormous ones. No matter what continent they settled in, be it the US, Europe or Australia the family breasts followed them. It was not so much a blessing but the family curse, although all the men in my life were rather partial to them and would beg to differ.

If I had to choose an animal totem for the female members of our clan, based on body shape, it would be a cross between a pigeon and bull. I guess that would make us the Pull or Bigeon tribe, so whichever way you look at it, regardless of feathers or hide, we are a big chested and proud lot. Luckily breasts make a comeback historically from time to time so if we are patient we're bound to be back in vogue soon.

Luckily the doctor didn't take out his sharp pincers to measure them because he would have ended up wearing them. To my absolute despair he announced after scanning my body through his glasses for several minutes that I was top heavy. Hello! Tell me something I don't know. I'm the one who has been hauling these beauties around for years, massaging the grooves in my shoulders and the pain in my back.

Another doctor, one who at least had enough humanity to share a good laugh, muttered that he couldn't hear my heartbeat. Basically my breasts got in the way and no amount of rearranging could get my heart in closer range. I had to admit to a moment of panic until the thumping in my chest reminded me that my heart was still there. Well protected from the barbs of man and just as loving as I remembered!

Don't you just love well meaning acquaintances who after years of watching your boobs sag down to your knees, offer a subtle suggestion? 'Have you ever thought about having a breast reduction?' they ask casually, as they grab a dim sim off the appetizer tray and down another glass of wine. Casually, so as not to offend.

'Thanks,' I reply. 'But I've already had one.' The satisfaction comes as I watch them skulk away embarrassed while I demolish the rest of the buffet. The frustration lies in the fact that after having my breasts cut down to size at an early age they just grew back again. They're just part of who I am and I have had to learn to accept it.

Back to the dreaded O word. Obese. Let's face it, it's ugly.

Obese. Tucked away in the dictionary alongside other horrible o words like obscene, obscure, obtuse, obliterate, oblivion, obstetrics, obnoxious and obsolete. Then there are others I'm not familiar with, like obfuscate … to darken the mind; obloquy … public shame, abuse and discredit (I rest my case), obsequies … funeral ceremonies and not to forget … obituaries. Not a pretty bunch.

The synonyms for fat are equally as repellent. Words like stout, portly, heavy and corpulent. Corpulent! It sounds like an army of corpses standing to attention. Then there's flab, blubber and adipose tissue. Hurtful, slushy words more befitting an unfit whale. What about lard? Or chunky, thick, hefty, podgy, rotund, fleshy or enormous. These terms don't exactly have a poetic ring to them. Now let's try slim. Lean, slender, trim, taught and terrific. Get the drift and the obvious bias.

Back to obese. A word that is bandied around to explain every complaint and affliction known to mankind. Headaches, diabetes, gall stones, fallen arches, hangnail, yellow spots, fleshy overgrowth, global warming and fungus. Obviously fat people can't reach down to dry between their toes. What a cop out! Like the time one supercilious doctor advised me to breathe into a paper bag when I was gasping for my last breath. She showed me to the door and it's a wonder she didn't shout 'fatty' on the way out. A more thorough medic ordered an MRI and immediate surgery when a serious brain condition was discovered.

The arrogant doctor was one of those medics that attribute every woe of the human condition to weight. They are often too slack or short sighted to look deeper to the true cause of your ailment. Or they don't care enough to probe further, into the intricacies of your body and mind. Worse still they may be 'holier than thou' and totally unsympathetic to the measures you have already gone to to control your weight.

You already feel lousy about it so why add to the indignity? What about your spiritual health? Do doctors ever advise you just to be happy? Or understand that all the anguish you go through to shed just a few unwanted pounds adds up to a lifetime of unhappiness. Or weigh up how that frustration causes your emotional and psychic destruction, which will lead to a much quicker and more painful demise than the extra weight you are carrying. Shame, guilt, heartache and failure are much heavier burdens to carry than fat.

During my last consultation with my neurologist, just as I was getting up on the couch to be examined, he muttered, 'chocolate is not that good for you,' which I thought was rather an odd comment considering he was about to test my reflexes. Whether chocolate has been proved to diminish nerve responses was irrelevant. I was offended that he assumed I was addicted to the stuff. I checked my blouse and there were no leftover traces of a Snickers bar to give me away but rather a not so sweet assumption. That my size was the result of being a closet chocoholic, and the cause of all my pumped up nerve endings.

I was angered on a number of levels. On a personal level and on a moral one. While waiting to see the doctor I had spoken to a young woman in the room outside. She looked wounded and had given up trying to control her crying toddler. When I asked if she was alright, she gazed into the distance and replied. 'I woke up a few weeks ago to find that I was blind in one eye. Scans showed a white spot on my brain and I have been diagnosed with multiple sclerosis.'

When I suggested she join a support group to help her through her pain, she turned away unable to handle her potential deterioration. 'No, I don't want to know.' When I passed her on the way out I wanted to scream, 'Eat more chocolate. Lots and lots of it.' What I really meant to say was to enjoy her life while she could. Bask in the sunlight and the joy, enjoy the pleasures of the earth while she was still able to.

When a friend's mother was put into a nursing home and could no longer eat, she was kept alive by a tube feeding sustenance into her body. She pleaded with her daughter to end it. 'Why stay alive when there is nothing left to enjoy?' she argued and in many ways she was right. To exist is not enough, one must LIVE.

Obese is a word that shoots you down in flames. I take exception to the label, as one specialist referred to me in his medical report. He used the word dispassionately as if it was a hair color or blood type. I have never felt obese. My friends assure me that I'm not, scoffing at the mere suggestion. I have no trouble sitting in an airplane seat and am comfortable at the movies. I only take up one seat on the bus, so why?

The term is simply based on a number or staunch figures on a scale. If the BMI is used as a yardstick most of the population would be considered obese. Not for a moment did the doctor take into account my bone structure, my hereditary, my birth date or the fact that I was the smallest person in my family. How come this stranger felt the need to degrade me, especially after a mere thirty minute consultation?

Invariably the doctors who condemn you are no picture of shining health themselves. The female medic who recommended the paper bag was one of these rangy lean women with bones that looked like they were forged in steel. Her face was so hard that a smile would have caused a hairline fracture. The specialist looked worn out and dull, and a naturopath I went to see had the worst case of dandruff. How am I supposed to trust these people with my health, especially when I look far healthier than any of them?

A word of wisdom for all those who have been shamed because of their weight. Thin people get all the regular ailments too, along with brittle bones, arthritis, and nasty wrinkles. Not to mention strange looking veins that wrap around their extremities like clinging vines because there's no flesh left to pad them out. Think of all those air brushed celebrities with arms that look like roadmaps that lead to all fifty states of the US. What's more thin folk also get fungus like the rest of us because their skin becomes so taut that mould gets in the cracks.

Overweight is another dreaded O word. It's not quite as vicious as obese but just as misleading. Overweight? Over whose weight? A leading Japanese sushi chef? A Tongan weightlifter? A Slavic grave digger? A Chinese contortionist? Or just me.

The subject of my first lecture in Psychology 1 was, 'What is normal?' Did normal refer to the norm, what most people did even if that behavior was abnormal or abhorrent? If that was the case then the sixty percent of the population who carry too much weight are the norm. They are normal. The skinny lot who are poorly represented are way outside the box and therefore should be considered abnormal. There obviously is no correct answer just as there can be no ideal weight. Thin people have their own cross to bear, some cannot for the life of them put on weight no matter how hard they try. However their body issues are generally not classed as detrimental or unacceptable.

While I was standing at my local railway station one day I noticed a poster on the platform warning of the dangers of crossing the lines. Splashed across it was the message that a train weighed considerably more than the average person of 129 pounds. I nearly threw myself onto the railway line in despair. Was my heavy weight enough to stop a charging locomotive, stop it dead in its tracks while others were scattered to the wind?

One day while tracing my ancestral roots I found a rare photo of my father's family that was sent to us from Greece. In sepia tints sat several generations of the family in all their glory. There was not a smile among them which was understandable as they were a hefty lot and obviously had to have all their clothes especially made. My mother's family are Hungarian and also came from big boned, glorious stock. And I am proud to be like them, big hearted and bold.

One of my 'groan' expressions used to describe someone of slender appearance is 'they're blessed with good genes.' Excuse me. I come from a family of doctors and philanthropists that date back to the tribe of King David. My great, great, great grandfather was so esteemed he was appointed physician to the sultan of the Ottoman Empire and my mother speaks seven languages and is a member of Mensa.

However I supposedly have 'bad' genes because they're a little fatty round the edges! I don't think so. What about those people whose body springs back into shape after childbirth like a malleable rubber duck, or doesn't alter after birth control, hysterectomy, menopause or giving birth to several offspring. Something doesn't quite add up here.

Even a tree gets bigger every year, with the number of rings on its trunk a measure of its magnitude. It shows how many seasons it has lasted on the earth and how they have left their mark. With each year the tree increases in both size and strength. Its roots become more firmly planted in the ground. Shrubs flourish with time, flowers blossom but some people show no visible sign of growth. Go figure.

Here are some disturbing facts to contemplate.

1. The average woman thinks about her weight every fifteen minutes and wishes she could be 30 pounds lighter.

If only we had something more pressing on our mind. It's a sad reflection of our society that our thinking is so preoccupied with our looks. Or that we are obviously so averse to our own self image that we are determined to alter it at any cost. Is our world so shallow that we cannot find a place for ourselves in it, exactly as we are?

2. Many women who now present with the onset of anorexia are in their mid forties. In fact 40% of women with eating disorders are mature age, with one doctor's patient presenting at the age of 68! Aren't the golden years the ones where you get to call the shots and enjoy life? Why is our society so narrow minded that it pressures us to conform to the point of being miserable and why would you be so submissive at an age when you should be standing up for your rights?

It's the 'Desperate Housewives' syndrome with shows that set impossible standards and turn decent beautiful women into desperately unhappy souls. It manifests not only in extreme purging but in equally debilitating behavior, such as guilt about eating fattening food, constant weighing with moods being determined by the whim of the scales and the incessant counting of calories and carbs.

The irony lies in our perception of beauty. Women lap up shows like Sex in the City and its slender fashion conscious stars. Sarah Jessica Parker is a favorite in her designer clothes and sky scraper shoes which would send the lesser of our species reeling down the stairs of the local subway station, ending up in a heap under a speeding train. However Sarah was recently labeled by a men's magazine as the least attractive of women which begs the question of taste.

Men obviously view beauty differently than women who are brainwashed into believing that they must be reed thin to be attractive. Many men prefer voluptuous women and personal preference dictates what type of woman they are attracted to. Men too can succumb to the expected image of what constitutes a hunk, with great abs and pecs.

I watched horrified as one male on a TV current affairs program placed himself on a beer diet. His diet consisted solely of beer and a few crackers and Vegemite to soak up all the fermented hops. He lost weight but was also rapidly losing his mind which he considered preferable to being 'a fat pig.' At least the girls liked him now that he was thin, stoned and impoverished. Or so he thought.

I refuse to be victimized because I was born round. There's something infinitely beautiful about the curve of an arch, or the arch of a curve. There are also some splendid applications of O. O is round and luscious. O stands for opulent, oasis, ocean, ornate, open, original, optimist, opalescent, oracle, orchestral, opportunity, Olympian, omniscient, orgasm, oxygen and lastly, oneself. Celebrations of life. O also stands for one of the most influential women in the world. Oprah.

Self to Oprah. In my humble opinion you were put on this earth not to prompt people, or yourself, to shrink and become less than they are but to inspire others to celebrate how they were created and grow towards the light. To promote a wondrous acceptance of self that has sadly been denied to far too many for far too long. What greater inspiration can there be? There is great wisdom locked in the planets and the higher truths of the universe will set us free.

One last word on O. When you slash O and let out some of the pressure as you would the air in a balloon, you are left with C. So obese then becomes cuddly and curvaceous. Whip C into shape and you get S. Sexy, sultry and sensuous. It's all a matter of perspective and your self image can be altered with one stroke of the pen and a fresh outlook on life. ALWAYS REMEMBER TO BE PROUD OF WHO YOU ARE AND TO LIVE YOUR MOST AUTHENTIC LIFE.

FOOD, GLORIOUS FOOD

'Nothing would be more tiresome than eating if God had not made it a pleasure as well as a necessity.' Voltaire

Are we wrong to enjoy food? To savor its heady aroma, smooth textures and divine taste. I think not. Even the gods were not immune to its delights. The food of the gods was ambrosia which was carried to Mt. Olympus on the wings of doves while smooth nectar was their preferred drink. Both were fragrant enough to be used as perfume and conferred ageless immortality. Sweet, delicious and good for you.

For us mere mortals, chocolate is the 'food of the gods'. Olmec Indians were the first to grow cocoa beans between 1500-400 BC. The Mayans made a drink out of it but its enjoyment was restricted to the elite. In the 14th century it became popular with the Aztec upper classes who called it xocalat. Chocolate was prized even then, by a privileged few. Over the ages, chocolate has been recognized as special.

The explorer Cortez made mention of it but it was not till Dominican friars took a contingent of Mayan nobles to visit Prince Phillip of Spain that it appeared in Europe. They brought a gift jar of beaten chocolate for the king, ready to drink. He was so smitten that Spain and Portugal guarded their treasure closely, refusing to export any of their beloved drink to the rest of Europe for nearly a century.

It was the making of a guilty pleasure. The Spanish added sugar and flavorings and by 1570 chocolate had gained popularity as a medicine and aphrodisiac. The first chocolate house opened in London in 1657, and as it was expensive it was considered a beverage for the elite class. Lucky Cadbury's came along and made if affordable.

Then there is ice cream which can be traced back to the 4th century BC. Early references contend that the Roman Emperor Nero ordered ice to be brought down from the mountain and mixed with fruit toppings. A gift from the heavens, it truly was 'food of the gods'. King Tang of Shang, China, created an iced milk concoction and after adding some syrup and sprinkles you have the birth of the ice cream sundae!

The Eskimo Pie ice cream was created by a shop owner in Iowa, USA in 1920, prompted by a young customer who was obviously a Libran and couldn't make up his mind between a chocolate bar and an ice cream. So the shop owner covered the ice cream with chocolate and eventually put it on a stick. A genius move and very lucrative too.

If you have a savory tooth, you'll be interested in the origin of popcorn. Known as 'prairie gold' it made a lot of farmers rich. A funeral urn in Mexico about 300 AD depicts a maize god with symbols of primitive popcorn on his head. Ancient corn poppers, shallow vessels with holes in the top, were found in pre Inca Peru so those folk obviously enjoyed munching on popped corn while watching sunset over the step pyramids, or the mass slaughter of sacrificial virgins.

The Native Americans brought popcorn to the English colonists as a token of goodwill during peace negotiations. Who wants tobacco when you can have popcorn? According to Indian folk lore, inside each corn kernel lives a quiet, contented spirit. When heated by the sun, they become angry until they burst out in an irritated puff of steam.

During World War 2, most sugar in the United States was sent to the troops on the frontline so there was little left behind to make candy. To compensate Americans ate three times more popcorn than normal. With the advent of television in the 1950's there was a sudden rise in popcorn sales by 500%. So began the pattern of crunch and watch.

Just for the record, it was Native American George Crum who invented the potato chip in 1853. He was a chef at a resort in the US when the mega rich George Vanderbilt came in to dine. The millionaire complained that his French fries were too thick and the rest is history. Lays took over, and with packaging came the start of an empire.

To appreciate the importance of the humble spud, we only have to look to the potato famine that occurred in Ireland between 1845 and 1852. When the potato crop in the country continuously failed because of a pathogenic water mould that was known as potato blight, there was widespread devastation. This was followed by typhoid, cholera and starvation that reduced the total population of the country by 20%. It may be only a lowly potato but it has the power to save a nation.

Although it is popular belief that the Venetian merchant Marco Polo brought spaghetti to Italy from China, it's not true. Pasta was already recorded in Italy from the 1st century AD, with noodles that were called lagane, lasagna nowadays. They were baked rather than boiled but no doubt just as appetizing because the Italians have a knack for cooking delicious fare. Add a lime gelato to cleanse the palate.

It was not until the 19th century that pasta met tomato. Even though tomatoes were brought back to Europe after the discovery of the New World, it was a long time before they were considered edible. Even back then there was a healthy distrust of anything that was good for you. A member of the nightshade family, rumors abounded they were poisonous. Eventually they were accepted and the Greeks turned them into a great salad by adding some black olives and feta cheese.

Finally let's discuss the iconic Coca Cola, and raise a glass to toast its remarkable success. The original Coke drink contained nine milligrams of cocaine per glass which may well have accounted for its popularity. The original stimulant was mixed in by way of coca leaves from South America and imported kola nuts provided the caffeine.

The trademark curvy shape of its bottle was said to be modeled on the contour of a cocoa tree seed pod. Others claimed it was inspired by the hoops of a Victorian dress. A famed designer stated that it was 'the most perfectly inspired package in the world.' The song 'Coca Cola Shape, Dat Sexy Body Remix' says it all. Following recent body trends its packaging has scaled down from curved and sensual to thin and sleek, and it's nowhere near as inspiring.

These foods and drinks are addictive because simply stated, 'they taste good'. For centuries these indulgences have been the domain of the elite and for the most part only royalty and high classes could partake of their pleasures. They were out of reach of ordinary men but now they are as close as the supermarket shelf. No longer are we deprived of these treasures but we do need to use common sense.

A friend explained one day over lunch that as a child she felt she missed out because her family were not well off and they never went out to dinner nor could they afford any treats when she was growing up. As soon as she was old enough to earn her own living she indulged herself on whatever food her heart desired. It was the ultimate blessing, to enjoy nature's bounty but she went overboard and paid the price.

These days it's not easy. We are given so many mixed messages. Buy low fat or skim milk, or better still soya. The next day, 'the risks of soya?' What about butter or margarine, popular opinion switching every week? We are barraged with products that are reduced in cholesterol, ones endorsed by the heart foundation, packaged goods with healthy names and a long list of artificial ingredients that can only be deciphered with a magnifying glass. How are we supposed to keep up or not be confused? Is there anything out there still safe enough to eat?

The US sprays two billion pounds of pesticides each year on its crops. These poisons end up inside our bodies which are incapable of eradicating them. In packaged foods there are chemicals used to color, emulsify, stabilize, bleach and texture food. The FDA lists about 2800 international food additives and 3000 chemicals in food products. These overwork our organs and saturate our cells, and can only be detrimental to our health and general wellbeing.

One friend of mine developed chronic fatigue syndrome, as have many people over the last decades. Her generalized body pain left her debilitated and the doctors could not help. She and her husband had once owned an organic winery in country Australia, and her symptoms began when the apple orchard next to their property crop dusted, spraying its fruit with strong pesticides. She suffered the after effects. An unnatural process, our bodies are not meant for such a barrage.

From an early age we are subconsciously programmed with sayings about food. Ironically the foods that are supposedly good for you cop a beating. The egg comes off the worst. 'He's a bad egg', 'to egg them on', 'to have egg on your face' or 'to walk on eggshells'. I don't know what the egg did to deserve such a shady reputation but it's being punished now with a high cholesterol reading, once again by eggheads and eggsperts who confuse rather than inform us. If I was a hen I'd watch out before you end up being genetically modified to lay eggs without a yolk for the frothy in-set who like their eggs beaten not stirred.

Comfort foods scores better because they make us feel good. 'It's a piece of cake' and a task couldn't be easier. Success is certain when things 'sell like hot cakes'. 'Butter wouldn't melt in her mouth,' or 'it's as easy as pie.' We love our sweets. 'When life hands you lemons, make lemonade,' implying that just a little sugar will make it alright. We all need a little sweetening. We show our love with terms of endearment like 'Sweetie, sugar, honey.' If we admire someone we say that 'she's a sweetheart' or 'she's a peach', or 'as sweet as apple pie', although I would avoid calling anyone a tart, a fruit loop or a nutcase.

Thin food doesn't fare well in comparison. 'He's bitter and twisted', or 'has a sour temper,' is not so good. The saying, 'as cool as a cucumber,' indicates veggies are not considered the sympathetic type, nor are they an especially active lot when you can become 'a couch potato'. I fondly recall on first arriving in Asia being told by several men in an attempt to woo me that, 'we may be small but we're hot like chili!' Being averse to chili the words did not have the desired effect.

We have even taken to naming our offspring after sweet ripened fruit, charmers like Peaches, Cherry, Apple and Plum. Thankfully the trend has not rippled across to vegetables, because some poor child would end up being named Beetroot, Turnip or Leek. Mind you Cubby Broccoli fared well and grew up to produce James Bond Movies. While tracing my family tree I discovered a distant auntie named Sultana and am most grateful that I wasn't named after her.

Back to the sayings. 'As keen as mustard' and 'to bring home the bacon,' appeal to the more savory types but who can beat the all time favorite, 'Cheese!' Think of a full bodied cheddar or a pungent blue vein so that you can smile for the camera when you find yourself surrounded by a group of dreadful strangers and are suffering from a hangover. Traditionally pumpkins are used at Halloween but they're pretty scary. Bugs Bunny loved his carrots, and spinach made Popeye big and strong so he could deck the dim witted Brutus and capture the heart of anorexic Olive Oyl. Olive is not a good role model. She must have lived solely on a diet of pitted olives and spinach leaves to get so thin and raspy.

We are told fruit is good for us but it may come to us disguised. 'An apple a day keeps the doctor away' but look what happened to Snow White. One bite from that tainted apple and only a prince could save her. How tantalizing it looked, how bright and shiny and beckoning, but it was riddled with poison and almost led to her demise. Not to mention Adam and Eve but that's another story.

Apples and other fruit can remain in frozen storage for seven months before they actually reach you. Knowing that we still prefer to buy them, rather than the organic variety which looks less perfect. It says something of the human mind that we judge quality by the outside appearance in more ways than one.

The irony is that the fruit has to be round and juicy to attract us because it appears to be brimming with life and nutrients. We are not drawn to the thin, mangled, mottled variety. Rather we like fat, shiny, perfect fruit. Its very sight can plump up our health and replenish our spirits. So perk up. Remember that 'life is just a bowl of cherries.' Lie back and enjoy it, preferably with someone who can peel you a grape!

THE FAT EPIDEMIC

Every day we are barraged with gloomy predictions about the obesity epidemic sweeping the world. Obesity is edging ahead of smoking as the number one cause of death, or so it is claimed. These dire warnings are interspersed with news reports of food shortages that are also sweeping the globe, with images of rioting in Haiti and African nations as food prices soar. Drought, flooding, plagues of insects, failed crops, have upped the ante as we have learnt to value food even more.

Food is life giving and essential to our existence. But there *can* be too much of a good thing and obesity *is* a growing problem. To add to the problem is the large amount of conflicting information and misleading reports about the subject. A recent newspaper article I read stated that the United States was the most obese country in the world, followed by Mexico, Greece, Australia and the United Kingdom. My heart missed a beat, being an Australian citizen who was born in Greece and British by marriage. I had bought a pot once in Mexico and love Hawaii so I knew I was cursed with the 'fat gene'.

Wrong. While researching the subject I was amazed to find what appeared to be several 'different' fat lists. The doctored version serves to scare all of us flabby members of the Western world and is no doubt compiled for that very purpose. Then there's the truer version. A recent report by the World Health Organization proclaimed that there were more than 1.6 billion overweight or obese people in the world. That's one heck of a lot of fatties so there has to be more to this.

Here's a surprise. Heading the trusted Forbes list with the highest level of obesity in the world is Nauru where 95% of the population are overweight. You may well ask, 'Exactly where is Nauru'? Let's just say if you were flying over the Pacific Ocean and blinked you'd miss it. Nauru is the world's smallest republic and occupies only eight and half squares miles. The smallest nation with the largest people. Go figure.

Presumably these people have no fast food outlets to blame their girth on, so what's going on? Look at the broader picture. Next on the list is the Federated States of Micronesia, then the Cook Islands, Tonga, Samoa and several other islands I've never heard of, where obesity levels are well over 80%. In fact the Pacific islands account for the top seven in the fat list so there's a lesson to be learned here.

Studies have been carried out on these islands to explain why the majority of people are overweight but most came up with lame excuses. 'These people once had a traditional lifestyle based on agriculture and fishing and now their staples have been replaced by rice, sugar, flour, and canned meat.' Much too simplistic. Most of Asia subsists on a diet of rice and it supports some of the leanest people in the world.

Accounts by early European visitors to Nauru noted, 'Nauruans are a plump race who admire big fat people. They put girls on a diet to fatten them up to make them more attractive.' I know this is a stretch but can we concede that these people are actually meant to be big, as part of the whale clan or 'people of the ocean'. Pacific Islanders have big bones and strong powerful physiques which they are proud of. It's probable with the consumption of refined food that they have gotten bigger but they were never a small race of people to begin with.

What's more they admire 'big'. Like a number of diverse cultures, they perceive big as a symbol of abundance and beauty. I once watched a documentary set on one Pacific Island where the bride of the chief was stuck in a bamboo cage and force fed so she would be even more attractive. It's not a method I recommend although I'd be tempted to lock a few Hollywood starlets in there with her, to plump them up with some taro root. In Africa there is a society where fat women are the cream of the crop and are so valued they are allowed the choice of husbands and take more than one to satisfy them. Polyandry at its best.

Now here's an interesting statistic. After the top seven island nations on the 'big' list, in sneaks the rich Middle Eastern country of

Kuwait at number eight, edging out America into ninth place. 74% of Kuwait's population are chubby, so it gives you some idea of what these folk are spending up on. The very best life has to offer. Food.

The USA then thunders in at number nine on an ice cream high, followed by several Caribbean nations with loads of bananas and then Argentina no doubt because of all their beef. It is trailed by Egypt with too many falafels, Malta and Greece with their love of olives and New Zealanders who are partial to sheep. Australia comes in at twenty one with a glut of health and muesli bars and even Mongolia rates a mention at thirty four, so they must be lapping up the yak butter milkshakes.

One of the few Asian countries to be included is Indonesia which streaks in at forty four. There seems little reason for this as their diet doesn't vary much from the rest of the Asian continent. Granted the people do like their food but have you ever seen the way lean Chinese plough into food in Singapore or Hong Kong, where they're spoiled for choice? Apart from their love of shopping, these races are definitely not the athletic type. Yet they remain thin, with no plausible explanation.

Could the determining factor be their genetic makeup and the fact that each race is essentially created as different? Just like the orangutans that roam the Indonesian jungles of Kalimantan, each animal species is unique and irreplaceable. 'Orang' means person and 'hutan' is the jungle. These 'people of the jungle' are a distinct species, just as people are meant to be. Distinctive, unique and special.

In affluent countries where there is a glut of food that is as delicious as it is tempting, there are hidden traps that often warp good judgment. These may result in overeating and a perverted self image. Morbid obesity is not an original state of being. A person who has descended into this state has allowed their inner balance to be sorely disrupted, just as an anorexic or bulimic who purges their food.

Morbid obesity and anorexia are eating disorders, and both are extreme cries for help. The body image has been distorted and unable to synthesize their outer appearance with their inner state these people fragment. Food becomes a weapon of destruction, used to cut the ego up into sharp, jagged pieces. Like a jigsaw, these pieces must be put together again so that a clear picture of the self can be obtained and healthy integration can take place. Of the mind, body and soul.

There are many reasons why we overeat, or chose to deprive ourselves with drastic diets. Most often it's a self depreciating backlash against what society has conditioned us to believe is attractive. We are presented with a so called 'ideal' and when we don't match it we become disheartened and disillusioned. This conditioning begins at an early age, when a puny or plump child is programmed to believe they are not good enough because they don't conform to an accepted image.

They don't belong in fairy tales and they don't have happy endings. They may be maligned and called nasty names, or constantly put down. They are rarely the star of the high school musical nor are they on the cheerleading squad. They are not the center of attention and are not voted the prom king or queen. They may not even score a partner, or be invited. If they do, more than likely their dress will have to be made because they can't buy anything decent off the rack.

This negative pattern continues throughout life. I was a chubby child who grew into a plump adult. I was not exceptionally large but I may as well have been a leper in my society. In a large city like Sydney I could not find anything to wear. Over the years some stores eventually put in larger sizes, albeit begrudgingly judging by their drab styles. Many of the clothes were shapeless and unflattering and they made me feel just the same. So I went in search of something to wear that would make me feel attractive but I always returned home empty handed and broken hearted. Others I met on my quest were equally depressed.

I met one such lady while in a tortured position in front of a store mirror. I had managed to stretch a jersey top over my bust but now it had me in a stranglehold for having the audacity to try it on and refused to let go. This nice lady helped me escape its clutches, while explaining that she was out shopping for her daughter. Or at least trying. Since her daughter had put on weight after having her first child, she refused to go shopping. She had tried several times to find clothes to fit but would always go home in tears. How demoralizing.

She was fortunate to have only suffered for a short time but worse still, she knew what she was missing. What about those people who have never been spoiled or felt desirable? No wonder they're depressed having been cast aside by society and made to feel invisible or unworthy. No wonder they resort to food to comfort them because it's one of the few things left for them to enjoy. To top it off, they're made to feel guilty about that too. Every other pleasure has been taken away so why not take away the last one too. Total deprivation.

In a defiant backlash, the more fragile of these oppressed folk turn their back on food altogether or else eat themselves into oblivion. Repressed, they can no longer venture outside their homes which to them is a relief as they no longer want to deal with a harsh world. They have succeeded in becoming truly invisible. If others turn away and pretend they're not there then they too can refuse to see themselves.

Even now when almost half of Western people are a plus size, shopping is still a chore. Several good stores and designers have risen to the challenge but some malls still do not have one single store for plus sizes, and in those that do you are lucky to get one or two shops for them compared to the scores of others that are designed for the spoilt slim lot. Do the math. If fifty to sixty percent of the population are plus size why aren't the same percentage of the stores catering to them.

The prejudice is obvious. 'Where are your plus sizes?' I ask as I enter a large department store, a question I am loathe to ask in case there are none or I am immediately branded a desperate fatty. Invariably the shop girl answers, 'In the corner, at the back.' As if the store is trying to hide its large stock under a bushel, as well as your fading light. As you swish past racks of fabulous designer labels for the rake thin, you are met with a paltry display of outfits more suited to the matron of a bowling club or as curtains for your sunroom.

So you are forced to retreat to the back of the store to sift through the retailer's pathetic attempt to appease their larger customers. Deflated you return home empty handed and resort to the internet to surf the World Wide Web to try to find something to wear. As I said, invisible. You don't have the luxury to try on the clothes, you just have to take pot luck and hope for the best. It's just not good enough.

Such is the bias that exists in our society that a friend with a plump teenage daughter told me that her daughter refuses to go into the only trendy store in the mall for plus sizes even though the clothes look good and fit her. She is so horrified that her friends will see her inside that she prefers to suffer in clothes bought elsewhere even though she can hardly breathe let alone do up the zipper on the outfit.

Try finding something to wear at a charity shop which is a perfect example of the skew that exists. The entire display is mostly small sizes with a few motley coat hangers with the leftovers of some poor large soul who has more than likely passed away recently. So rare are plus sizes it's very unlikely that anyone in their right mind would give up an outfit once they'd actually found it. It's a stinging indictment.

Then there are large size bras, more suited for the military, with enough metal underwire to repel a shrapnel attack. They could be recycled to work as bulletproof vests or to test airport alarm systems. It's hard enough having to lug hefty breasts around without a tortuous apparatus designed to stop you breathing. Craftily most stores put their large bras at the bottom of the rack so you have to stoop down real low to get to them. It's a good ploy and they'll make you exercise yet!

I have travelled the globe and always had trouble finding clothes to fit. Some countries like the USA are more progressive but others are way behind. Understandably having lived in Asia for a while made it more difficult but what about a place like Singapore? Supposedly it's the shopping capital of the world but try to find any clothes of a reasonable size! There are plenty of large sized women living there, not to mention tourists but no go. The large majority simply don't exist.

It's a lose-lose situation. Why do stores and boutiques restrict their clientele to thin people when they only have to cut the cloth larger, to go to normal, average or plus sizes? Wouldn't they at least double their profits if they expanded? Isn't that what we call good business sense? Are they so bloody minded and shallow that they think large people don't deserve to look good or that their divine fashions will be compromised on a larger body? It's all part of some warped conspiracy.

Those wretched little designers have a lot to answer for or else all the clothes are made in a village in China where they've never seen a large person in their lives. One day when I was in the jungle in Nepal on an elephant walk, we chanced upon a tiger. It was such a rare sighting that several elephants, carrying enthralled guests on their backs, circled the tiger. The tiger took one look at all those elephants and was out of there. He jumped so high, he leapt right over one of the elephant's heads! Absolutely no doubt, they're threatened by us.

Now look at all the images that confront us every day. Ads that show slim supple beauties who deserve to have the world thrown at their feet. Fabulous jewelry and lingerie while us larger folk don't even warrant a watch. Some straps, made in the same factory in China no doubt, don't even fit around my wrist. In any case if you're big you don't need to tell the time because you obviously have nowhere to go! Who would want to go on a date, or dine, with a fat wristed woman?

It's my ultimate dream to see billboards splashed across the mall showing curvaceous women wearing tiaras and diamantes, with adoring males groveling at their feet. I yearn for a grand poster of Fabio swashbuckling across the deck of a pirate ship, clutching a Rubenesque wench in blue jeans by his side. Better still, she could tie him to a pole and have her pick of the rest of the crew. What's more I want to see her eating a rich gelato, and licking her lips in ecstasy.

I want to see that it's OK. That it's OK to be big. That big means beautiful, plentiful and enticing. I need to remember that large equals abundance and that voluptuous Venus is the goddess of beauty and she loves life. I want to be reminded of my own beauty, a hazy image that has been erased over the decades by default or be misguided intention. More than anything else, I need to know that it's OK to be me.

IT'S ALL A PLOT

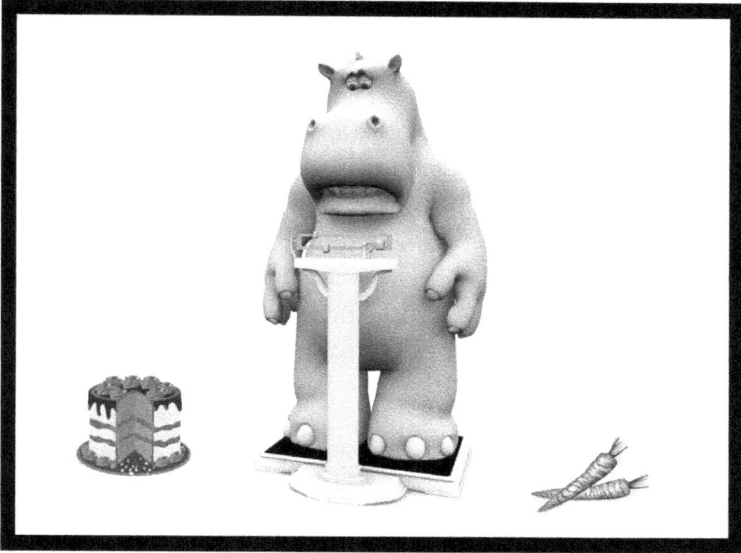

Something's not quite right here and I smell a rat. It came to me while watching a rerun of the movie My Big Fat Greek Wedding last night. What a happy bunch the Greeks are as compared to the staid Anglo Saxons. I should know. I was born in Greece and married a nice British man. The Greeks are a festive bunch who like to make a lot of noise and socialize compared to the Anglos who are rather a restrained race in comparison. The Greeks also love to eat. Probably why they made it into the big five in the 'fictitious' fat list, ironically along with the stoic Brits and Americans, the sleepy Mexicans and the sporty Aussies.

After a lot of thought I sprang into action. I was confused so I felt compelled to trawl the internet to set myself straight. As one of the top five so-called fatties in the world the whole Greek race is doomed if all the prophecies are right, and fat will lead to their ultimate demise. In a strange twist, earlier that night I watched a program extolling the value of the Mediterranean diet which the Greeks created. All that lovely fresh Greek salad, rich black olives and goat's cheese and yoghurt was apparently the key to leading a healthy life and to losing weight.

Here's my confusion. Aren't the Greeks eating their own diet? Absolutely and they're loving every tasty morsel. They may well be piling on the calories with a few late night baklavas and kouribedes cookies but they easily burn those off by chucking a few plates against the wall and dancing wildly in circles. Could it be this atrocious truth ... that they're fat and healthy? If the statistics showing Greece has the lowest incidence of bowel cancer in the world are to be believed, then yes. An impossible truth. They're chubby, healthy and happy.

With my curiosity piqued I popped onto Google searching for answers to the puzzle that has confounded man in modern times to the point of madness. I wanted to discover whether fat was really the determining factor to longevity. What I found out confused me even more. None of it makes any sense, if we believe everything we are fed. In my opinion it's our minds that need to diet. It was only fitting I find the answer on an American CIA list because the whole thing smacks of a global conspiracy. The CIA list referred to the Country Comparison of Life Expectancy at Birth, the average number of years a person born in a certain place can expect to live. Life expectancy is also a measure of 'overall quality of life in a country and summarizes its mortality.'

Small places rate well where perhaps the pressures are fewer. Number one on the list is the gambling capital of Macau in China where you can expect to live to 84.36 years on average if you can afford to live that long. In second place is the tiny European principality of Andorra, nestled between France and Spain, where the fresh mountain air works its magic. Coming in third is Japan where all those years of eating raw fish finally pay off and then a close finish between Singapore and Hong Kong where you can apparently shop yourself into a long life.

The first 'large' country to enter the picture at number six is the land down under, Australia with a median age of 81.63. Now correct me if I'm wrong but wasn't Australia in the top five fatty list. So how come they're not all falling off the face of the planet instead of topping the longevity list? Something doesn't add up here, especially since they just squeeze out the French who work hard at being slim, svelte and sophisticated. The Aussies outlive the French by almost a year, so 'French Women Don't Get Fat' but Aussies do and live longer.

It seems to be a strange trend, this 'chubby power.' Tubby Greeks come in at number twenty six on the list beating the tall rangy Danes who enter the picture at number forty five. So all those lean cold cuts might seem good for you but shortbread dusted in icing sugar is better. All those years spent bicycling in the cold can't beat dancing in circles after drinking too much ouzo by the light of a big bright Aegean moon, clutching onto the arm of your new best friend.

The USA is a bit of a worry, trundling onto the list at an unimpressive forty nine, just ahead of Albania. In a major world power we expect a better performance but with a failing health system, food portions better suited to a tribe than an individual and a disproportionate number of morbidly obese people, some of whom are so overweight a building has to be demolished in order to get them out, then this is an issue that needs to be urgently addressed. It's important not to confuse overindulgence with wealth or with deprivation for that matter. The rich deprive themselves so they can be thin while folk in deprived countries eat more to feel wealthy.

Now let's look at number one on the true fat list, Nauru. Along with Kiribati and Vanuatu, is doesn't do so well at number one hundred and sixty eight on the life expectancy list with the average life span at just 64.20. In real terms it beats out nearly all of the African countries where people are thin, impoverished and suffering from disease. Last on the list at two hundred and twenty plus are Zambia and Angola. There people only live to 38.20 years. So it seems fat folk outlive thin ones in real terms, for fat exists in countries where there is a glut rather than a famine. At the end of the day that is always preferable.

Now let's take a look at another list, one compiled by the International Living Magazine which attempts to quantify the *quality* of life and the best places to live in the world. According to them a number of factors determine the top places to live out of a possible one hundred and ninety contenders. These include the cost of living, environment, health, infrastructure, safety, climate, culture and leisure.

Now here's an interesting overlap. Number one on the list for five years in a row is France, narrowly beating out Australia in second place for the gold ribbon of fabulous life style. The two major nations that competed for the highest life expectancy also have the best quality of life. That's no surprise. So perhaps the key to a long life is very simple after all, *happiness*. A good place to live, then expect a long life.

Both the French and the Australians know how to enjoy themselves. The French revel in their culture, love their art and go for long walks along the Seine. The Aussies revel in their culture, love their art and go for a brisk surf or swim on the beach. They also share a love of good food. The French are famous for their cuisine, fine wine and delicious pastries. The Aussies have lashings of good, wholesome food, fine wine and tasty treats. It's all about attitude. To quote the magazine on its selection, 'I wish the quality of life indicators could measure a country's heart and soul.' Quite possibly they do. It's all about believing that you have a right to a good life, enjoying the best life has to offer while finding and maintaining a healthy balance.

Now here's an interesting comparison on a personal level. My mother is a big, beautiful Hungarian woman and as a Gemini she loves to read. I remember as a child watching as she retreated each evening into the lounge room for some 'me time' with a book in hand and a jar of goodies. For her nothing beat nibbling on a handful of nuts while reading a science fiction classic or one of her favorite authors.

Two of her best friends were sisters, French by birth. Both were slim and obsessed with their weight. One talked about it incessantly to the point of boredom and only allowed herself small portions of yoghurt or cheese so that she could fit into her designer clothes. The other was fanatical, walked for miles each day and ate only a little grilled meat and vegetables, which she prepared for herself each day.

Tragedy came in their later years. The first sister developed Alzheimer's disease and is scarcely coherent on a good day. If research is to be believed and brain cells must be used to reduce the risk of developing this debilitating disease, then the mind has a greater purpose than to count calories and to shop for the latest designer outfit. Of course some very astute people have fallen victim to this crippling disease so its onset and cause is as baffling as it is heartbreaking.

Despite her strict 'optimum' life style, the second sister was diagnosed with pancreatic cancer and passed away within a few weeks. Sadly she never allowed herself any sweets and *to my mind* denying the pancreas its function, to break down sugar, is just as lethal as overloading it. As I said, it's all about finding the right balance.

One of my favorite sayings states that no pleasure is worth giving up just to spend a few extra years in the geriatric ward. Why on earth would you want to prolong your life if you're not enjoying it? Every day when I walk to the station I pass a home for the elderly, a hospital of sorts for those dear old souls who can no longer look after themselves. Much to my distress I hear the same old man call out each time I pass, with the same desperate words. 'Let me out of here,' he screams over and over and my heart pangs a little each time I hear it.

What a dreadful fate. We humans face inordinate challenges every day, some minor while others can be soul destroying. To sweeten the load we have to allow ourselves pleasure, the riches that this planet has to offer and afford our lives a touch of bliss. In moderation but with joy and gratitude, we have to appreciate all of life's treasures so at the end of our days we can look back with happiness and contentment.

YOU ARE
WHAT YOU EAT

Ludicrous statement: **YOU ARE WHAT YOU EAT**

If that was the case then only cannibals would be human because they eat other people.

Stupid premise: **YOU ARE WHAT YOU EAT**

I love sweets. Heaven is full of chocolate éclairs and ice cream and dreamland has mountains made of lamingtons (sponge cake dipped in chocolate and flaked in coconut) and rivers of crème brulee. According to the premise, I must be sweet. It's actually true, except when someone stands outside my apartment at 3am bellowing into their mobile phone with a voice that reverberates all the way to New Delhi. I get so annoyed I yell a lot and then retreat to the comfort of my kitchen to find something sweet to eat so that I can become sweet yet again.

Most Watched TV program: **THE BIGGEST LOSER**

In the guise of offering them salvation, a group of flabby people are divided into teams to compete in the eternal battle of the bulge. They are starved and then forced to do push ups or other such athletic tortures, including such indignities as pulling a heavy locomotive along a track like a team of oppressed pack mules, almost giving themselves a hernia or heart attack in the process. We already know fat people are branded as losers so why rub salt into the wounds? The contestants are urged on to the point of belittlement by well oiled trainers, who yell abuse as a form of 'encouragement'. Personally I'd like to feed these trainers to the sharks but with so little meat on the bone and all gristle, the sharks would probably chuck them back onto the boats.

Doesn't this whole scenario remind you of a 'fat witch' hunt or a zesty day in a Roman arena, when Christians were being fed to the lions? All the courtiers eating grapes with their thumbs down, sealing the doomed one's fate. However in those days it was the fat ones who were in charge. Do I sense a hint of revenge? Now if Sophia Loren walked into the ring, I'm guessing it would have been a thumbs up from the crowd. If it were some of the emaciated starlets of today, I suspect even the lions would have turned and walked away in disgust.

Strange Irony:

The most popular program on Aussie TV, apart from the grand final of some sporting event, is Masterchef. This fabulous program pits one hopeful chef against another as they melt saucepan loads of butter, roast shanks of pork and drip Grand Marnier sauce teasingly onto a warm sumptuous chocolate pudding. Then drizzle some icing sugar or plump berries over the top for added effect. Stomachs rumble and taste buds salivate all across the continent in one collective groan.

The next top rating program after Masterchef is the Biggest Loser shown on the same network. Now I'm no rocket scientist but even I can see the connection. You rush out to the supermarket so you can cook all the wonderful recipes and then you spend the next few weeks trying to get rid of the backlog. The missing step between cooking and purging is EATING. Don't encourage us to eat and then belittle us for doing so.

Some people with miraculous metabolisms do get away with it. Most of the competing chefs in Masterchef fall into this category, remaining thin by either burning off all the calories in their dash from the oven to the bench or because they never get time to actually eat any of their creations. Fortunately last year's winner had the satisfied happy look of someone who actually enjoys her meals, just like the delectable Nigella Lawson. It's hard to vote for a lean mean chef who seems at odds with the very concept of the blissful place food can take you.

Ridiculous TV program:

Picture this shocking scenario. Some poor soul has the weekly contents of their stomach spread out on their dining room table for the whole world to see. Six cartons of fried chicken, hot and spicy, four boxes of Donut King donuts with chocolate sprinkles, eight hamburgers with the works, with extra pickles and large french fries. Then there's the dozen bottles of cola that are corroding their intestines as we speak.

Despicable. The whole world condemns them for their folly. Can this misguided person not contain their animalistic urges to gorge and stuff themselves with the fodder of the 21st century? Where are the artichokes and asparagus, the lettuce leaves and crisp endives? Giving over to the collective will, this poor misguided fool allows some mean looking woman, eerily reminiscent of the Wicked Witch of the West, to strip his cupboards of anything that even remotely resembles food in a last desperate bid to 'save' him. He is then placed on a stringent diet of boiled radishes and turnip greens.

Meanwhile some unfortunate person who is aptly named 'crash test dummy' is forced to eat all the junk that the fatty has been piling into his body in a sadistic effort to show just how bad it is for you. They fold within a matter of days, illustrating just how diabolical the diet is. Even more gruesome is the fact that they undertake such a task in the first place, being such a radical departure from their original diet.

This was especially the case when one dummy (I mean this quite literally) drank copious cans of energy drink laced with caffeine each day plus black coffees with very little food to soak it up with in order to mimic the crazed habits of one of the participants. It's a wonder she didn't end up dying from the effort or at least running berserk and butchering the Wicked Witch with a can opener, or the show's director.

While there is no doubt that a fat person may well have created their own misery by overindulging in a shameful diet of diabolic proportion, we are left with one very disturbing fact. The false assumption that thin people are saint-like because they curb their animal urges and eat well. Instead here is the truly shocking reality.

FOR ONE FAT PERSON WHO EATS ALL THIS STUFF, I'LL SHOW YOU TEN SKINNY ONES WHO EAT JUST AS MUCH IF NOT MORE!! THEY JUST BURN IT OFF BETTER.

Why are we fed this rubbish? Not the food, the lie. Why is the truth not exposed? That some of the population can eat anything and get away with it. They burn it off with the ferocity of a furnace fuelled by turbulent DNA. After serious research, like hanging around outside Baker's Delight and Wendy's ice cream parlor, I made a startling discovery. The majority of customers were thin. They were choosing to stuff calories into their mouths without a thought or a shred of guilt while some unfortunate plump person hovered in the background, holding back from the rest. Depriving themselves because they had been shamed into it or were frightened of the consequences. Sob.

Here's another biting reality. FOR ONE FAT PERSON WHO EATS A LOT I'LL SHOW YOU TEN OTHERS WHO EAT VERY LITTLE. MUCH LESS THAN THEIR THIN COUNTERPARTS.

Continuing in the vein of good research I checked out a number of fast food outlets and was surprised by what I saw. Without a doubt, thin people order more giant servings and larger portions than stubbier folk. More big Macs, burgers with the works and overflowing dishes of whatever takes their fancy. My findings were confirmed at Subway where ninety percent of the orders for foot long bread rolls stuffed with juicy meatballs and similar, were ordered by the thinner customers. Plumper people mostly ordered the six inch roll with leaner cuts.

If you don't believe it, check it out for yourself and it may just turn some of your perceptions around. We are so used to mindless images of large people stuffing themselves with food that we take it for granted even though it is often far from the truth. I know from my own experience that I don't eat much compared to others. I can barely scrape up an oatmeal breakfast and whenever I buy takeaway for lunch I throw half of it away through loss of interest or lack of appetite. Granted I graze at night, but purposely have little in the cupboard to excite me so that I am not tempted to stray. I don't drink alcohol, don't smoke, don't indulge in soft drinks, don't drink coffee and don't put sugar or milk in my tea. I don't eat red meat. There's a lot of don'ts there.

Far too many to make any sense. Consider a typical day at the supermarket. Here's how it goes. I dutifully fill my trolley with bottles of mineral water and strawberries, tomatoes and fresh shiny things. Then off to the frozen section for a pile of microwave diet meals. Fine tuna in basil, salmon shanks in brine and other oil bearing flesh. Omega something or other. Then I come to aisle three. The danger aisle.

It's stacked with biscuits and chocolates. My hand reaches over towards my favorite Swiss block and then trembles with a conflicting mix of longing and trepidation. In one daring move, like a ravenous snake striking at its prey, I grab it and throw it in my trolley. By aisle five however, I am racked with guilt and hide the chocolate among a stack of toilet tissues chastising myself for being so weak.

The supermarket is littered with treats that have been foregone by repentant dieters in a pang of conscience. Others do not understand the pain of such dismal deprivation. One day while gazing longingly at the chocolate marshmallow biscuits, a reed thin grand dame of eighty, boasted that she ate a large TIN, not a packet, of chocolate Tim Tam biscuits each night. I wanted to pummel her to death with the metal lid.

Which leads us to the faulty equation.

THE FAULTY EQUATION

If I was being totally honest I'd have to admit to a wayward childhood. When I was two years old my family migrated to Australia from Europe and my parents bought a toy shop. It fuelled my fantasies and my imagination ran riot among all the dolls and fairies. My favorite was a bride doll, dazzling in her white wedding gown that stood just out of reach on the top shelf. Instead I ended up with a dusky island girl with hoop earrings and a straw hula skirt. She may have been a symbol of my later love affair with the islands and their beautiful people.

After several years my parents sold up the toy shop and bought a grocery store instead. In one corner was a big wooden tub for the bread. As you know, the aroma of freshly baked dough is far too tempting to resist. To make matters worse biscuits came in large tins in those days and the selected amount weighed and placed in a brown paper bag.

Unfortunately little hands could reach into the tins and abscond with some of the spoils. I spent many afternoons after school sitting at the counter munching on a warm bun, or on an Iced Vo Vo biscuit or Adora Cream Wafer, while reading the latest edition of the True Confessions magazine. What more could a young girl ask for than being immersed in a romantic tale while nibbling on a fresh roll or sweet treat.

An even more sordid confession is what my sister and I would get up to late at night. We would take turns at creeping down the stairs, after our parents had gone to sleep, to dip into the glass chocolate cabinet. Then we would return with our ill gotten gains, stealing back up the stairs and into the bedroom. What a treasure! A handful of fizzy treats, with insides the color of a rainbow. Or a packet of chewy toffees or a yummy Kit Kat bar. We even had our secret hiding place, a loose floorboard in our bedroom to hide all the wrappers. It was only years later that my father chanced upon our naughty little secret. Until today he complains that's where all his profits went!

When I was six years old I got lost among the masses of people at the Royal Easter Show. I wandered off among the cow stalls and the prize winning rams, searching for my animal totem, oblivious to my parent's panic as they searched everywhere for me. Eventually they tracked me down in the police tent, where I was enjoying an ice cream cone surrounded by a group of policemen. This accounted for my later love of comfort food and men in uniform, an irresistible combination!

It's hard to shake a habit, especially one that you love. Some people can get away with indulgence and remain slim while others pay the price. There is no pat formula as to why some folk get to eat what they want while others are forced to restrict and deny themselves. Nor is it a simple equation of food equals weight. We are indoctrinated with the idea that if we cut our food intake and exercise, we will lose weight. A simple mathematical formula, but is it?

I wish it was that easy. For the last twenty years I have divided much of my time between Sydney and Bali. The diets of both places are diametrically opposite. The Western diet is more wheat orientated, with many more sweets and refined carbohydrates. Bali has a spicy Asian diet, with boiled rice, meat and fresh vegetables as the staple.

While in Bali, I stuck to the Asian diet especially in the early days when little else was available. I never developed a taste for chili, but otherwise I ate like a local. In both countries I enjoyed fresh fruit daily although Bali had a lot more tropical varieties. Even though I ate more calories in Australia my weight rarely fluctuated. I was heavy in both countries and the restricted Asian diet did not promote any weight loss. Way back then in Bali there were no chocolates either.

Then there's my lovely friend, Lily, a singer from Sumatra. She is five foot nothing and usually struts around in shiny red stilettos and mini skirts. A wisp of a thing, she barely weighs more than a feather. But how that girl can eat! After Lily devoured four courses at lunch, she'd munch on a jumbo packet of chips on the way home while driving the car. I dare not even put one in my mouth. The packet of chips was bigger than Lily's body but she still managed to eat the lot. I wondered where it all went. Did she have some invisible chute in her head that catapulted her massive calorie consumption into space? It certainly wasn't anywhere to be seen on her tiny body.

Another case in point was my assistant in Bali. Ayu was in her thirties and had worked for me for many years. A quiet young lass, she was all bones and no flesh. One day she confided that she was desperate to put on weight. She ate constantly and even resorted to a special *jamu*, or local herbal cure, that had been specially mixed up for that purpose. Nothing worked. She came from a thin family and was a Capricorn.

Even though most Balinese are slim, some defy the rule. Access to my house in Bali is down a small pitted laneway in which lives a huge woman with ponderous breasts. There is not enough rice on the island to have made her so big but she seems unperturbed by it all. It was the custom in Bali for centuries for women to go topless and this woman sticks to it until this day. I think her reasons are less cultural but rather arise out of necessity. On this island of svelte dancers and slender maidens, the poor woman would never be able to find a bra that fit.

Recently I attended a meeting held by a naturopath on the island. The subject was weight loss and she had brought along two ladies to speak on the subject. Both were larger than the country's norm and had suffered the consequences. One had been big from birth and was teased at school about it until she developed a debilitating complex. The other had been a high fashion model in Jakarta in her twenties but over the past few years had piled on the weight. As Indonesians tend to be direct in speech she now suffered the cruel taunts of past acquaintances, who asked outright, 'Why you are so fat now?'

Not only did the unfortunate woman have to bear the anguish of a large weight gain but also the relentless onslaught to her ego. So the cycle escalated and even though her weight gain had been primarily caused by hormonal changes she began to eat more to spite her critics. Here's the deal. FAT HAPPENS. Don't chastise yourself over it as if you have committed some unpardonable sin. It's just part of life.

If you're still not convinced about the inconsistencies of weight let me tell you about my cats. One lived in Australia, the other in Bali. Both are Persians. My white Persian Abby in Bali is a female with a big appetite. She eats four meals a day but remains thin. I try to fatten her up with butter croissants and cheese, which she loves, but she never puts on weight. To this day she is light as a feather.

Whenever I bring something sweet home I have to hide it from her but Abby has a nose like a bloodhound and can smell it from a distance. After feeding her a nice plate of fish in the kitchen as a decoy, I skulk off into the bedroom to eat a cream cake. Within seconds Abby zooms in at the speed of light, clawing her way up my arm to get to the spoils. Forget the main course, let's have sweets! She just loves them.

Merlin on the other hand is a black Persian I once fostered in Australia. He was a rescue from the Cat Shelter and after I took him home he was so relieved he guzzled down food for a week. Then he found his balance and became fairly indifferent at meals. He ate twice a day, fairly small portions, but after several months he put on so much weight I almost got a hernia trying to pick him up. He was a stocky lad.

Now here's the poser. Both cats were fed the same brand of cat food, with the same size portions. Both got up to no more exercise than finding the best spot in the house to fall asleep in. However one was spayed and the other was not, one had been abused while the other was pampered from birth, they came from different genetic stock and were born in different months. These were the variables that explained the differences in their weight. Food and exercise were not the deciding factors.

Think about it. If you starve a Persian cat you will never get a Siamese. The cat would not morph from cute and tubby into sleek and angular. Nor would we want it to. I love the Persian's doll face, broad head and stocky legs. They say animals reflect their owners and that's exactly the point. We're all attractive in our own right. Take people with their dogs. Tall lean people often prefer the elongated breeds like Afghan hounds and greyhounds. Short people like Maltese terriers, bassett hounds, poodles and the like. Broad people seem to like St. Bernards or labradors, while a friend of mine had a bulldog that is the spitting image of her. I'm not game to say it to her face in case she sets Bluto on me!

We're all different, they're all different and in the end we match. That's the joy. Is it such a hard concept to grasp that some people, like animals, are meant to be bigger? That real variety is what makes our earth unique and interesting. We don't try and shrink our animals, unless we have overfed them, so what are we doing to our people?

As final proof of the faulty equation, I offer two graphic examples. The first was told to me by a friend who worked in a nursing home. There she tended to elderly people who could no longer care for themselves. The size of each person did not alter with age. One woman was so gaunt, her skin was like fragile eggshell. Another was so big it took four people to turn her on the bed. Both women had been in the nursing home for seven years. Both had eaten the same meals, with no treats in between. Both were bed ridden with no exercise. Yet both women retained their original body weight until the end of their days.

The thin one died years before the heavier one and despite all the forecasts of doom and gloom, my friend insisted it was most often the thin ones who passed away after a debilitating illness not the fat ones. The larger ones had the body reserves to fight back and survive. Yes, life is rarely predictable nor are the rules of existence cut and dried.

My final example makes not the slightest bit of sense and is definitive proof of the faulty equation. On the program Amazing Medical Stories was the baffling story of people who suffer from the malady of eating while they are sleepwalking. These people while asleep will get out of bed during the night to eat. They eat all manner of strange things, including soap, dog food sandwiches and other such yummy treats. They have no conscious understanding of what they are doing and have no recollection of it whatsoever when they awake.

One chubby lady was confused as to why she had put on 15lbs over the past six months even though she had not altered her diet, at least not on a waking level. Video surveillance revealed to her that she got up two times during the night to partake of a midnight snack and went back to bed still chewing her treats. The next morning she was baffled to find empty wrappers and the odd banana skin by her bed.

Now, here's the real teaser. Another young lady who suffered from the same condition since she was a child, according to her worried yet resigned parents, got up on average *ten* times during the night to eat. Despite going to bed continuously on a full stomach, this slim lass had not put on an ounce of extra weight despite her years of excessive binge eating. She remained slim despite her overindulgence in food. How on earth can we even begin to explain this phenomenon? It does not make sense, nor will it ever while we cling to that same old faulty equation.

IT'S WRITTEN IN THE STARS

If there's one thing I believe in implicitly it's the subject of astrology. It resonates on an instinctive level and has proved itself time and again in practice. When we come to realize that our passage is determined by the position of the planets at the time of our birth and as they transit in the sky, then even the most arduous experiences become enlightening as we learn to accept the wisdom of the universe. There *is* a divine plan.

The first time I consulted an astrologer I was not yet versed in the subject but was keenly interested. The astrologer painstakingly drew up my chart and then smiled. A wry, accepting smile. His words were not those I was hoping to hear. 'You weren't born to be thin,' he said, as tactfully as he could. What he actually meant was that I was born to be round but he wasn't game to say. 'You have all the abundant signs and planets prominently placed in your chart, a generous placement.'

Now I have nothing against abundance or generosity but I don't really want to be so blessed. Hoping he'd made a mistake I retreated to the bathroom to consider the subject. One look at the mirror set me straight. There was no doubt, I was born to be round. Later when I came to know astrology better I understood his reasoning. I have every hefty planet in the solar system placed prominently in my chart and if there is a goddess Fatty I am her reborn. To set the record straight, there are several elements in our horoscope that determine the way we look.

The first and most obvious is our Sun Sign. It's the sign we check in the newspaper each day, to see if we're about to self destruct or meet the love of our life and then self destruct. Sometimes our sign doesn't ring entirely true. When you're described as a horny Aries but you're heading for a nunnery to spend your life in contemplation and practice celibacy, there could be an element of doubt. That's because it's far more complicated than just the mere placement of the sun in your chart.

In our future nun's case this can be explained because the planets that move close to the Sun like Mercury, Venus or Mars are usually in the same sign as the Sun or in the closest sign on either side. Thus they temper the Sun's position and influence it greatly. So our Aries nun obviously had her other planets in the sign of Pisces, directly before it, which shows the need to transcend primal urges and pursue spirituality.

Then comes the Ascendant. This is the astrological sign that's on the horizon at the time of our birth. It changes approximately every two hours and stamps a mark of individuality onto our being. This sign is the strongest indicator of what we aspire to look like even though we may have been born in a different sign. It gives us the opportunity to change our look if it's at odds with our sun sign and we're peeved.

The Ascendant is where you get to call the shots. Your mum might have wanted a nice docile Cancerian but you had other ideas. She may have been pushing with all her might to expel you into the world but you were determined not to be the mooshy sort and hung in there for another two hours, held your breath and refused to emerge until Leo spun around. After all, you were born to be wild!

At first mum dressed you in flimsy lace and brushed your luscious locks with a downy brush but as soon as your Leo roared into life you dyed your hair red and buzzed it into a Mohawk or had hair extensions until your hair exploded like the mane of a lion that had just been electrocuted in the hair dryer socket. In a leopard skin mini skirt and dangling earrings, you climb up onto the counter of the local karaoke bar to belt out a few bars of Lambada while strutting your stuff. Then again you might be one of those nice shy Leos who ties your hair into a pony tail and falls asleep in a field of poppies.

The third variable in the chart that determines our looks is the moon. Its position in our chart affects our appearance as expressed through our emotions. It also signifies the presence of the mother in your chart. That is why a child's moon is often found in the mother's sun sign. The moon is sensitive, so if it's located in a fleshy sign you're pure mulch and prone to puffiness. My moon is in lavish Taurus where my mother has most of her planets. Moon in Taurus roughly translates that any hurtful encounter will be appeased by a plate of luscious hot scones and jam and like my mother I love my sweets.

The moon in Taurus is exalted, which means the moon is in its best position in this sign. Obviously the Almighty believed that scones and jam were the most beneficial way to soothe the injured soul. Much better than beating yourself up over it like an Aries moon who will challenge a rival to a round in the boxing ring to fight it out, or a Capricorn moon who will turn to ice rather than admit to any pain or a Cancer or Pisces moon who will sulk for ages and then self destruct.

As we are complicated creatures, making the subject of astrology just as complex, there are many variables to consider. If one of your personal planets like the Sun, Moon, Mercury, Venus and Mars is joined to one of the planetary big boys, or slow movers, like Jupiter, Saturn, Neptune, Uranus or Pluto, you're a dynamic soul. On a personal level you take on some of the characteristics of the stronger planet. For example, the moon joined to Neptune in the heavens at the time of your birth makes you a spiritual person. Being a watery planet Neptune also creates flab, making you a flabby spiritual person. Why the Almighty equated spiritual evolution with puffiness remains a mystery.

The sun or moon joined with Jupiter or Pluto makes for a heavy body. If it's any consolation people with these connections draw on the substantial power of the stronger planet and are endowed with a certain charisma, authority or magnetism that marks them out as special. I hit the jackpot when it came to heavyweights, with my Sun, Mercury and Neptune sitting on the Ascendant, all in curvy Libra. Venus was having a field day when I was born, not to mention the moon languishing in ample Taurus. If that wasn't enough I was born in the Chinese year of the Ox. Heavy Taurus bull meets hefty Chinese ox so I was deemed, or rather doomed, to be round.

Now I'm not one to complain but that's a bit rough. Why not an agile monkey or a frisky rabbit? I'd even settle for a dog or horse. No,

I scored good old reliable Ox, the heaviest of the lot. I'm supposed to be compatible with the rooster or snake but I can't stand all that crowing and slinking around, or small talk about how I need to shed a few pounds, so I'd grind both of them into the ground with my sturdy hoofs.

Now here's some valuable advice in case you're considering slimming with the stars. Going on the premise that WE EAT WHAT WE ARE rather than 'we are what we eat', I present the following culinary guide for each sign. They are essential tips to understand yourself better or in case you are taking someone out to dinner or have been invited to their house for Sunday lunch. To each of my friends mentioned, I wasn't watching while you were eating or taking notes.

ARIES is the sign of the Ram and is ruled by aggressive Mars. It should like grazing on greens but prefers eating its own kind. An Aries likes nothing more than a good barbecue with lamb roasting on the spit or a big chunk of beef. All washed down with a couple of beers. It's the first of the signs and therefore the most basic.

I had an Aries suitor once but we lasted only two weeks. A Chinese kung fu master, a born fighter, he gave packed daily classes to his eager initiates. I endured two dinners with him before I threw in the towel. Being a vegetarian it was more than I could bear to watch him gorge on his blood red steak, with the juices still running raw, with such primal lust. When he topped if off by filling his steaming hot coffee with chunks of melting ice, I was out of there!

TAURUS ruled by sensual Venus is the connoisseur of the zodiac. Taureans loves the good life, a gourmet meal of roast duck and truffles set out on a lace tablecloth with the finest silver and crystal glasses, preferably laid out on a marble Louis 14th inlaid table. Followed by a glass of good wine over a box of imported Belgian chocolates while reclining on a chaise lounge by a warm open fire.

I had a Taurean friend, Beverly, who I shared breast reduction operations with. It was her second attempt to reduce her assets being a buxom bull with a tiny waist. Her first job at the Darrell Lea Chocolate factory almost proved to be her downfall. Unable to help herself, it was one sweet for the conveyor belt and one for her. A chocoholic's delight.

GEMINIS ruled by the mind planet, Mercury, are an easily distracted fidgety lot and are generally poor eaters unless they have some planets in Taurus to plump them up, steady them and increase their appetite. They eat for half and their alter ego twin got the better end of the deal. They like their food simple with not much variety. Gemini rules the chest, so unfortunately the weaker of the sign resort to a good puff on a cigarette rather than bother to eat at all.

My friend Suzi was reed thin and with her pointed boots and black leather gear was a bit of a leftover from an earlier rocker era. During the day she'd duck outside for a smoke and scarcely ate at all. Dinner consisted of a packet of instant noodles mixed into some stir fry vegetables, which she would nibble on half heartedly. In any case, she couldn't sit still or concentrate long enough to enjoy her meal.

CANCER, the watery moon planet, rules the stomach and those born under the sign crave nothing more than simple comfort food. A bowl of hot potato and leek soup with crunchy bread and a slice of pumpkin pie will do the trick. They are not averse to dipping into the pot, so a steaming hot crab dish or thick clam chowder will also satisfy them. Anything to stop the stomach rumbling and provide some good old fashioned nourishment. They like nothing better than to cook up a nice home cooked meal for family and friends in the comfort of their warm, cozy home, preferably in the kitchen while they stir the pot.

LEOS ruled by the exuberant sun love to eat in style, with great pomp and circumstance surrounded by a band of doting admirers. They enjoy nothing better than sipping on a splendid glass of champagne in fluted glasses while they talk their way through a five course meal. The more expensive the better, as long as someone else is paying for it. They'll even make you feel grateful that you actually got to pay for them. Lobster Mornay is all the go and only the best will do.

VIRGOS, another Mercurial lot, are health nuts and if they're not they should be. Concerned with cleanliness and germs they'll wear rubber gloves to prepare food or to clean up. They swing wildly so they could either be vitamin junkies or total slobs. In their optimum health mode they're into berry yoghurt shakes, raw vegetable juices with wheat germ and seaweed floats. Otherwise they're junk food addicts and don't give a toss.

LIBRANS, touched by the beauty and grace of Venus, are sweeties, hence their love for anything sweet. They will go out shopping for flowers and scented candles, purchase a lovely box of chocolate bonbons and French pastries done up in ribbons, while actually forgetting to buy any food for dinner. Then they will procrastinate for the longest time before ringing up home delivery and lashing out on a pizza supreme with the works, or in a fit of conscience pop a diet meal, Fettuccine al Fungi or Stir Fry Chicken a la King, in the microwave.

SCORPIOS, ruled by the potent combination of Mars and Pluto, like it hot. They're partial to curries and spices. They'll try any meal as long as it's from some distant part of the globe, the more exotic the better. On any given night you'll find them in a Turkish kebab shop tossing pita bread, at a Japanese sushi house sampling raw fish or burning their palate on flaming hot chili dish at a Thai restaurant. They can also be a bit Goth so they're attracted to restaurants that are painted black and are decorated with bizarre voodoo memorabilia, or are blood red with a vampire theme complete with steaming hot bat soup on the menu.

SAGITTARIANS ruled by expansive Jupiter have simpler tastes but in greater portions. Nothing satisfies them more than a big beef, double cheese hamburger and chips or a good Sunday roast. Then you have the extreme fitness types who will crunch on a whole wheat muesli bar while they're out on their evening run unwilling to sacrifice the time to sit down long enough for a really good meal.

Most are not content to sprint alone so they often drag the poor unsuspecting family dog behind them on a leash or push a horrified infant in a stroller.

CAPRICORNS, ruled by stoic Saturn, are into nuts and grains and being the goaty type they like to graze but preferably at minimal cost. Down at the pub they've been known to stuff a few extra peanuts into their pockets for a future snack. They're very frugal in taste and even more miserly in the wallet. Many a millionaire with Capricorn Rising has taken lunch to their penthouse office in a paper bag. Preferably, a nice cheese sandwich with an apple or banana. No fancy stuff for them and if they must lash out they prefer to buy at Coles. They're especially keen on the red light specials so they can buy out of date goods at half the price!

AQUARIANS touched by eccentric Uranus keep their waif like figures by showing a marked disinterest in food. They'd eat a book if they could, followed by a computer generated dessert. Aquarians would be good in space because they'd enjoy eating the simulated meals. They would even analyze them to see if they were good for you. As distasteful as it seems they are not partial to sweets, as if those exquisite taste buds were expunged from their mouth at birth. They could reincarnate as robots or as a Microsoft programmer next time round.

PISCES is the fish sign of the zodiac ruled by sensitive Neptune. Gentle Pisceans like to drown their sorrows and wallow beneath the ocean. Have you ever heard the expression, 'drink like a fish'? Well fishes don't but Pisceans do. They soak up the spillage with an array of fresh seafood and nothing pleases them more than a platter of king prawns, clams and calamari. Some brethren straight out of the ocean washed down with something fizzy and preferably alcoholic.

My Piscean friend told me one day that she was heading off on a picnic with some friends. Being a romantic Libran, my thoughts turned to a lovely checked tablecloth decked out with loaves of fresh bread, rich cheeses and fresh fruit. Not to mention a lovely apple pie with lashings of fresh cream to finish off the day. When I asked what she was taking, she simply replied, 'a bottle of Vodka.' I rest my case.

Now if you're protesting that your sign doesn't sound remotely like you, remember that many factors influence a birth chart. All of the planets interweave to form a unique pattern to create the special person that you are, unlike any other being on the planet. Life is a complex mystery and we are each one of the parts that make up the whole.

A prime example of that unique essence is the magnanimous star Oprah Winfrey. She was born an Aquarian, a lean air sign, which accounts for her broad intellect and love of books. However at the time of her birth the sun was in exact conjunction with the planet Venus, within eight seconds of each other. Such a close connection endows her with the beauty of Venus, her pleasing womanly shape and a good appreciation for the finer things in life. Adding to the mix is Jupiter which is trine to the sun and Venus. The bountiful planet Jupiter gives her a compassionate, humanitarian nature and also ensures her mass appeal and guarantees her success. Jupiter is a plentiful planet in all aspects which accounts for her hearty appetite and her love of food.

Yes, astrology as a map of the universe is extremely complex and it mirrors the individuality of each person. Our looks, body shape, temperament, mentality and evolutionary stature are unique to every one of us and we each face our challenges as best we can, growing at our own rate. The daily movements of the planets trigger certain people to enter our lives and elicit situations that can assist in that growth.

Transits of the planet also affect us on a different level. They cause fluctuations in our weight through no fault of our own. When Jupiter, the corpulent planet, transits through the personal houses of your chart, you only need to chew on an onion ring to prompt a body fat revolution and a massive meltdown of the psyche. Your appetite increases as does your girth. To give you a better idea of how the planets influence us, I now present a guide to each one. I begin with the weighty planets in our solar system, Venus, Jupiter, Neptune, the Moon and Pluto. If you are born under their magnanimous glow then you are probably charismatic, humorous, powerful and most likely round or as I prefer to say, voluptuous just like me.

I'M YOUR VENUS

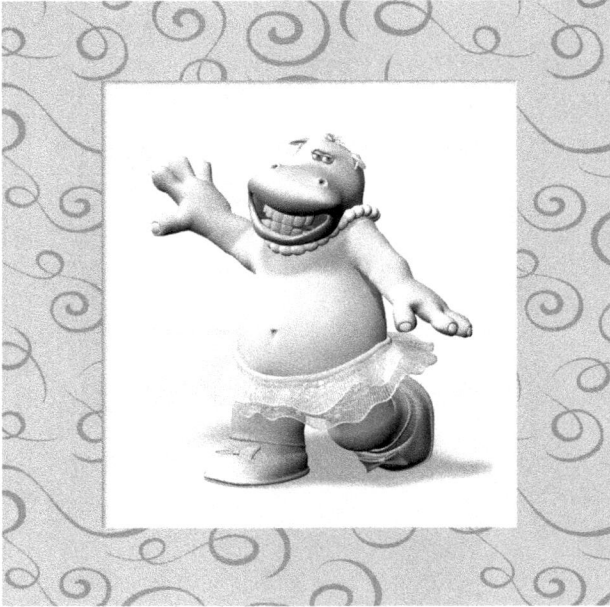

Ah, Venus the sweet goddess of love. How you have been immortalized over the ages! The Roman goddess of love, beauty and fertility, Venus was Aphrodite to the Greeks and was idolized. Just the way she likes it. Rather a self obsessed type, Venus craves adoration and devotion so she always has to look her best to ensure that she is the center of attention.

The classic painting 'The Birth of Venus' by the great Italian Renaissance artist Botticelli shows the goddess Venus rising up from the ocean on a fragile shell while angels bestow untold blessings upon her. Despite the wonderful imagery in the scene, Venus's conception according to mythology was not quite so ethereal or innocent.

Apparently Gaia, the Goddess of Mother Earth, was irritated at her husband Uranus for some transgression or other. It seems he was rather a playboy with a roving eye so he caused the goddess a lot of stress. She must have been really peeved in the end because she had his genitals sliced off and thrown into the sea. There they mixed with the foam of the ocean to create the wondrous Venus.

Probably because of the strange circumstances surrounding her conception, Venus was not one to stay at home and look after the kids. Far too concerned with having fun, Venus indulged in life's more basic and wicked pleasures. She reveled in her many affairs, one with bad boy Aries, or Mars the god of war, who put the excitement back into romance and another with the strikingly handsome Adonis. Being seen with the gorgeous young stud gave the goddess a welcome ego boost.

As Venus represents sensuality, beauty and pleasure, women who are born under her influence are the curvaceous, indulgent type. The placement of Venus in your horoscope indicates your approach to love and relationships and determines whether your affections are constant and deep or fickle and flirtatious. It also gives a clue to the hidden siren in a woman's chart, her inner goddess. In a man's chart it represents the type of woman he is turned on by, the sort to rock his world.

Even though you may not know the position of Venus in your horoscope you are sure to recognize aspects of yourself in the following list or the type of woman you may one day aspire to be. It will give you a guide to your office colleague's preferences and a head start when you're standing around bored at a party after work. You'll also know what you're up against when you're chatting up that cute guy at the bar. Happy hunting and may the best gal win!

Venus in Aries in a woman's chart indicates a bold aggressive type who will shove others out of the way if they get between her and the object of her desire. She may even hurl a javelin at you, so watch out and keep your distance. A man with an Aries Venus will like a woman with spunk, someone he can jump out of planes with or at least join the mile high club while still in flight. They're easily pleased and when it comes to lust they win hands down.

Venus in Taurus is much more sensual. She wants her partner to unfurl gold chocolate wrappers for her and feed her hazelnut creams with soft centers. He wants her to melt the chocolate on him and lick it off. They are the touchy feely types so once they have satisfied their desires he will arise from the bed and sculpt a perfect image of his love.

When placed in Gemini, Venus loves to talk. She will chat to her partner at all hours of the day and night on the phone and he will text message her while they're still talking. They will discuss every aspect of the relationship, play word games, do a crossword together, read a book side by side in bed and then discuss every aspect of it in detail. They'll even try to decipher the intricacies of the Karma Sutra before indulging because pleasure comes more from the mind than the body.

Venus in Cancer is a softie, an emotional sponge and a lover of Hallmark cards and Harlequin romances. It's the romantic fantasy that appeals to her but tread carefully because she is fragile. Easily hurt she will sob her heart out at the merest slight. He will console her by cooking up a gastronomic delight in the kitchen. They make a good match because she gets to cry while he's chopping onions.

Step out with Venus in Leo because she will definitely make her presence felt. This woman loves to shine in her bronze make up, killer nails and slinky sequined dress. If you want to impress her, take her to the theatre where she can imagine she is the star. He wants a diva, someone who exudes sex appeal and makes him feel grand.

Venus in Virgo are rather cold fish. They are prim and proper and will want a fully certified medical report before they sleep with you. She's good value if you want someone to organize your sock drawer and if you're a hoarder she'll sort you out pronto or add to the mess. He's a closet hypochondriac who wants a woman to take care of him and tend to his every need wearing a skimpy nurse's outfit and latex gloves. They either make a very sterile couple or a crumpled mess.

In Libra, Venus is in her own romantic sign and she's in her element. She will yearn to be serenaded under her window on a star filled night and to be read sonnets to, as he swears his undying love. She will expect him to forsake all others and swallow mandrake poison if he's ever foolish enough to stray. He worships his love goddess and keeps her on a pedestal where she belongs, all while strumming a lute.

Venus in Scorpio takes it one step further. She will slip cyanide in his coffee if he dare step out of line. A lethal mix of Mata Hari and Lucrezia di Borgia, she yearns for passion and intrigue and will not settle for anything less than the dramatic. He searches for a dark haired beauty reclining on mirrored cushions in an Arabian harem to whisk away on his smelly camel while offering her some Turkish Delight or a little exotic delight of his own!

The Venus Sagittarian will leap into her beloved's arms. She may bump into him while running a grueling marathon, swimming in the summer Olympics, literally bowl him over at a cricket match or topple over him in a bowling alley. He will have a thing for women on horses and will scour racecourses and police parades for his perfect match.

A chilly placement for Venus is in the earth sign of Capricorn. The original 'Material Girl' she is on the lookout for an octogenarian magnate who can shower her with Gucci bags and Prada accessories. A man who is on his way up in the world and preferably on his way out. She needs a guarantee that she will always be kept in the style she has become accustomed to. He wants her slim and perky, preferably synthetically enhanced, to be his glowing accessory. After all they both have an image to maintain and a reputation dripping with gold.

Venus Aquarians are quirky souls who will bump into each other in a rare and out of print comic shop, at the Museum of Technology, in the queue outside Apple awaiting the release of their new IPod or at a Star Wars convention. He will be dressed as Luke Skywalker and she will be Darth Vader. Theirs is an instant attraction that will endure even after they have taken off their costumes. It's a wacky Uranian thing.

Soppy Venus in Pisces will immortalize their love in poetry, in melodic odes that stand the test of time. He will be her Heathcliffe as they wander along the moors together thinking deep, destructive thoughts. Quoting Wordsworth, he will hand his beloved a freshly picked posy of daffodils while brushing aside the butterflies. Their love is so transcendent and pure, there's no need for base pleasures like sex.

Blessed are the people who are touched by Venus's hand. Libran women radiate beauty as the goddess works her magic through them. Perfect examples of her hour glass shape, lustrous hair and stunning good looks are the Libran actresses Rita Hayworth, Brigitte Bardot, Linda Darnell, Anita Ekberg, Kate Winslett, Catherine Zeta Jones, Mira Sorvino, Monica Belluci and Catherine Deneuve to name a few. The innocence of Venus shines through the radiant youthfulness of Julie Andrews and Olivia Newton John. The goddess likes to stay forever young and as a reflection of herself prefers her progeny to do so too.

Even in her men, the Venus charm prevails. It is reflected in the romantic ballads of Libran Julio Iglesias who can't stop singing of love's virtues and reputedly testing out its joys many times over for himself. She manifests in the suave panache of Roger Moore, Hugh Jackman, Guy Pearce, Michael Douglas, Viggo Mortenson and Matt Damon. In the penetrating beauty of John Lennon's music, the exquisiteness of Lucianno Pavorotti's voice and the poetry of TS Eliot. And the world is a better place for the beauty they bring to it.

There's an interesting story about an Australian swimming star of the early 1900's, Annette Kellerman, who illustrates the essential beauty of Venus. Annette lived an extraordinary life, as was recounted in the film Million Dollar Mermaid where she was portrayed by the lovely actress Esther Williams. As a young child Annette suffered from a weakness in her legs and they were placed into a painful brace to strengthen them. Hoping to improve her condition, her parents enrolled Annette in a swimming class. It proved not only to be her salvation as she became stronger, but also her great passion. Annette went on to win several swimming medals and was the first woman to attempt to swim the English Channel. She tried three times but was unsuccessful. Hoping instead for a career in movies, Annette made several films that featured her skill in precision swimming and diving. They were aptly named Venus of the South Seas and Neptune's Daughter.

With her perfect body and her skimpily designed swimwear, scandalous at the time of billowy dresses that trailed into the water, Annette caused quite a stir. A nasty incident saw one couple in court after the wife attacked her husband with a potato masher after he went to see her movie a staggering three times! She probably had her Venus in Scorpio and couldn't help herself. In 1908 after completing a study of 3000 women, a Dr. Sargent of Harvard University dubbed Annette the 'perfect woman'. He found her measurements to be exactly those of the famous statue of the Venus de Milo, the personification of beauty. Annette turned out to be an exact replica of her form.

Her Venus influence was written in the stars. When Annette was born, Venus formed a perfect angle with Jupiter in the sky, in the sign of Libra. Indeed Annette was the embodiment of the goddess Venus. The sign of Taurus is also ruled by Venus but in this placement her influence manifests more in a desire to be surrounded by beautiful things and to collect fabulous objects. It is a strong feminine sign. Queen Elizabeth of England is a perfect example. As a Taurean not only has she ruled over her country for decades but her wealth is astounding. Not to mention her jewelry collection which is to die for!

From the earliest times Venus has been represented as fecund and ripe. Hers was the beauty of abundance and fertility. Many great artists like Titian, Rubens and Renoir represented women as voluptuous and alluring and the marble statues of ancient times celebrate her as sensual and curvaceous. The captivating Mona Lisa is not your typical beauty and her enigmatic smile that has sparked people's curiosity over centuries has yet to be deciphered. But it's obvious. Either she's just scoffed down a steaming platter of cannelloni behind Leonardo's back or hidden the vanilla slices at the bottom of the cupboard where he'll never find them! She's a woman with a secret and we're intrigued.

Singers are not oblivious to the charms of Venus. They have sung of her beauty since olden times and over the years she has been found on the top of a mountain, in blue jeans and in Billy Idol's thoughts. Unfortunately she has been transformed into plastic Barbie Venus and how we do her an injustice. More than anything the goddess knows that true beauty comes from within to glow on the outside. Venus is the brightest object in the night sky so learn from her and shine your light. True beauty comes from recognizing your radiance and basking in its glory. Just like the goddess you were born to shine.

BY JUPITER

Jupiter is a bountiful planet, one that confers good fortune and success. The largest planet in the solar system, Jupiter contains more matter than all of the other planets of the solar system combined. It enjoys being a heavyweight, circled by a rim of colorful latitudinal bands and twenty eight satellites. Its atmosphere is deep as are those born under its influence. They understand the value of learning and higher education.

Because of its mushy gaseous interior, landing on Jupiter would be like immersing yourself in a cloud of marshmallow. Your 'soft place to land.' This positive planet makes everything all right and buffers every ordeal with a guardian angel and a happy ending. However Jupiter can be a hard taskmaster and the planet's storm clouds come complete with lightning bolts. In his original form Jupiter was Zeus, the king of the gods in Greek mythology. He ruled over Mt. Olympus and was known to hurl a few bolts of his own. Zeus loved to dish out punishment to the mere mortals below, dispensing good and evil from the jars that were placed beside the gates of his palace. Zeus protected the innocent and punished murderers and other wrong doers.

The Romans turned Zeus into Jupiter, their prime god who ruled over law and social order. The deliverer of cosmic justice, he was also known as Jove. In ancient Rome people swore honesty to him in a court of law and from that practice we get the expression, 'By Jove.'

Jupiter brings with him abundance and wisdom. The colors associated with Jupiter reflect his status - imperial purple, violet and indigo. When Jupiter's influence is strong in a birthchart we find persons who are both learned and astute. They may hold positions as judges, lawyers, teachers, clerics and religious scholars. Because these people are knowledgeable they can be heavy in build, indicating their firm grounding. Hence the expression, 'his words carried weight.' Defined by the dictionary, 'weight indicates a degree of importance and great influence as in 'arguments of great weight' or 'considerations that hold great weight.'

Famous Sagittarians, the sign ruled by Jupiter, include Winston Churchill (no lightweight, in any sense of the word), Charles De Gaulle, Mahara Ji, Mark Twain, Louisa May Alcott and George Eliot. Their words carried weight and influenced many with their thoughts.

Interestingly from Jove comes the word jovial, to be merry and full of fun. The inference here is to be truly wise one must have a good sense of humor and appreciate the inconsistencies of life. Jupiter people are generally an optimistic lot who love to laugh and enjoy life. If Jupiter is misplaced, they may enjoy life a little too much. Strongly placed in a person's chart Jupiter shows a tendency for over-indulgence and a probable past life as a gourmand or at least a French pastry chef. Being a weighty planet, anyone born under its heavy influence may carry some excess baggage, in the form of body fat.

To lighten the load, Jupiter loves a good belly laugh. This sense of humor inspires comedians, many of whom are heavy set. Most recognize the folly of their own predicament and love to laugh at themselves and poke fun at the rest of society for its short-sightedness. They see the divine irony, for when it comes to the tricky subjects of tolerance and acceptance we still have a long way to go.

Jupiter is also extremely generous. He likes to share his good fortune and so you may receive gifts for being a good sort. With a well placed Jupiter you're the lucky type who wins the lottery several times over. Others might not share your euphoria unless you share your bounty and make them happy too. Generous gestures in shows like the Secret Millionaire and Random Acts of Kindness are pure Jupiter. As for the big-hearted man who was giving away free hugs, I suspect Venus had a hand in that. She had little to show after the flower power love-ins of the sixties dried up so she joined forces with Jupiter.

The epitome of Jupiter's generosity manifests in TV quiz shows. 'Show me how clever you are,' Jupiter boasts, 'and I'll reward you.' The god is having a field day masquerading as a TV host and giving away heaps of money to those he deems merit it. First one has to earn it either by being diabolically clever or just plain lucky. Jupiter rules luck and those who have a perverse placement of the planet will be the world's worst gamblers and will lose both their pants and their dignity.

When we talk about humor and generosity, the most shining example of both is the greatest of all Jupiter archetypes. His rotund shape is typical of one whose Sun is linked with Jupiter at the time of their birth. He is the kindest and most big hearted person of them all, the one who brings joy to more people in the world than any other.

Who else but Santa Claus? He is virtually bursting out of his bright red costume with goodwill and cheer as he sings and chuckles his ways across the skies pulled by his band of equally jolly reindeers, Prancer, Dancer and the like. Merrily on their way. Santa's only mission in life is to bring joy and good tidings to the hearts of children all over the world. Celebrated on the 25th December, Christmas just inches over from Jupiter ruled Sagittarius to wily Capricorn because after all the merry making and gift giving, Saturn, its ruler, makes you pay for the lot and to budget and go without for the rest of the year.

Santa is a loveable, bespectacled man who is jolly and round. Could you imagine if Santa was thin and his clothes were hanging off him? If he slid down the chimney and landed in one of the socks hanging above the fireplace unnoticed. Unthinkable. Round is soft, wonderful, tubby, protective and nurturing. It shows a generous spirit, one that is brimming with life and abundance. That's why a child takes a teddy bear to bed to cuddle and not a giraffe. Ho ho ho.

Have you noticed that no one ever asks what Santa eats and how he got to be that fat in the first place? Has he been feasting on too many Xmas cookies and dipping far too often into the egg nog? Is it all those yummy snacks left out for him in homes across the world as he delivers his gifts and shares his joy? Dare anyone suggest he go on a diet and shed those unwanted pounds? No. Why? Because we love him that way, etched in all his chubby glory in the hearts and minds of adults and children alike from one far off part of the globe to the other.

When I lived in a country town and worked as a counselor, I was asked to be Santa Claus for the children's picnic. The rest of the staff were an emaciated lot and I was the closest they had to being jolly. The psychologist, who was a shallow egotistical lass with a fine figure, got to play my elf. I had a wonderful time being happy until I nearly wiped out a child while ringing my bell. It was hard to see behind my beard and I would have much preferred to aim for the psychologist. Ho hum.

And while we're thinking elevated thoughts, here's something to ponder. Buddha went off to meditate for seven weeks under a Bodhi tree in Nepal, without any food and water. He was on a Jupiter head trip and wanted to know the meaning of life so that he could teach it to his fellow man. He must have been down to nothing at the end, living on spiritual sustenance alone. All skin and bone and scrawny to boot.

However have you noticed that most Buddha statues are fat and smiling? There are few lean and gaunt images of him, strained from the physical sacrifice. Buddha went through many stages in his life but it seems that he is best loved in his happy rotund form. It seems most people equate nirvana and enlightenment with celebration of life and happiness. Not deprivation and pain or for that matter ethereal bliss.

When Jupiter transits through the twelve houses that make up your birthchart it brings the blessings of pleasure and abundance in the area that each house rules. When it moves through your second house you rush out to buy quality furniture so that you can surround yourself with luxury. In the third you will read a lot to expand your mind. In the fourth there will be joy in the home and in the fifth perhaps an addition to the family. In the sixth your health will improve and in the seventh Jupiter brings happiness in relationships. You may well meet the person of your dreams and they will treat you with the respect you deserve.

As Jupiter moves into the eighth house you develop an interest in the metaphysical or perhaps receive an inheritance and in the ninth you blow it all on travel to broaden your horizons. In the tenth house you take on a new course of study or receive acknowledgement or improve your skills. The eleventh brings support from friends and acquaintances and when Jupiter passes through the twelfth you will probably leave everything behind to go and meditate under a tree like Buddha.

There is great order in the universe and everything has its time to flourish. Jupiter wants you to indulge in the best life has to offer and get your just desserts. When the mighty planet hits your Ascendant, the sign on the horizon when you were born, and travels into your first house it brings you just that. Just desserts and plenty of them. Suddenly your appetite increases and you want to indulge in food to the extreme. You experience flavors you never dreamed as your taste buds spring into life and food takes on a whole new dimension. You indulge in new culinary delights in gourmet restaurants with a group of willing friends. As your appetite increases so does your waistline and your credit card bills.

If Jupiter creates stress aspects with other planets while it travels through the first house then you may pack on the pounds in spite of yourself. You may not have altered your diet but the weight still piles on. I know it's unfair but there's a perverse sort of wisdom in the universe, one of which I have yet to entirely master. Unfortunately Jupiter can take some time to pass through a sign or a house so you may be stuck with a weight issue that can stay with you for a lifetime.

If it's any consolation when stern Saturn comes through it may rip the pounds right off of you. Recently I had Jupiter move through my first house and my girth expanded as did my passion for sweets. Then along came Saturn a year or so later. As it hit its mark, its starting point in my chart in Virgo which rules digestion, I came down with a severe case of food poisoning. Saturn is no light weight and it hovered in the skies over this critical point for almost a year causing me havoc.

My gut felt as if it had been twisted inside out and I was so ill I completely lost my appetite. I made more loo stops during that time than I dare count and no amount of medication could stem the flow. I was worn out, miserable and defeated. Just the way Saturn likes it, challenging you ever step of the way. Worst of all, I lost my passion for food. It tasted bland and unappealing and I had to force

93

myself to take mouthfuls of soup. Bit by bit my body started to fall apart. The doctors said it was some nasty bug they couldn't identify and hopefully over time it would work its way out of my system. I knew better. It was Saturn causing me grief and I counted the days until it passed to leave me in peace. The interesting twist to this tale was people's reactions to my distress. 'I haven't eaten for months,' I confided, pale and drained.

'Oh, at least you will have lost some weight,' they invariably replied, reminding me of the silver lining to my tale of woe. It didn't matter that my body was slowly giving way. No at least I was thinner.

They say you can never be too rich or too thin. Rich perhaps, if you take Jupiter's advice and spend it wisely. Thin, no. You can be *too* thin if you're anorexic and no longer able to recognize a healthy image of yourself or if you're bulimic and try and purge that image from your consciousness. You may be too thin if you are sick or undergoing therapy which causes your body to deteriorate and waste away or if you live in an impoverished country and are slowly starving to death or are being deprived because of dreadful circumstance or nature's cruel whims.

What a terrible state of thinking if 'thin' is our top priority. Yes, I did lose a lot of weight but I would take it back in a heartbeat in exchange for my love of life and hearty appetite. To enjoy life once more and all the pleasures it has to offer. Even though one is supposed to be healthier when lighter I felt the opposite. I looked gaunt and my inner spark was missing. Things are not always as they seem and Jupiter's blessings are as rare as they are prized so learn to value them.

WATERLOGGED
THE MOON AND NEPTUNE

Plagued by cellulite? Or lumps and unsightly creases on your wobbly bits or arms that flap with the first breeze ready for take off? Blame it on the planets. There are two major planets that regulate fluids on the earth's surface, the tides of the ocean and other cycles. As humans we are composed of approximately sixty percent water so we are just as susceptible to their effects. As a result there is no way to rub or massage unwanted fluid out of your system or banish it away with creams or potions. Just go with the flow.

The moon is the first of the watery planets. In Greek mythology Selene, Phoebe and Artemis are the lunar deities while in Roman mythology the moon was ruled by Luna. It's only fitting that these are female goddesses because the moon's twenty eight day orbit coincides with the woman's menstrual cycle. The moon's ruling sign Cancer is the reason we often get 'crabby' at that time of the month and cause the men in our life to run for cover and like a crab, go hide under a rock.

The words 'lunacy', 'lunatic' and 'loony' all derive from the goddess Luna, all states that can be achieved by gazing at the moon too long when feeling melancholic. Admissions to mental institutions peak at the time of the full moon as does the crime rate so the sight of the glowing orb either sends you over the edge or off to rob and pillage. An astute nurse in the US found that the incidence of gastric hemorrhage and post-operative bleeding increased at the time of the full moon so the doctor's surgery schedule was arranged accordingly for the best outcome and the patient's recovery rate escalated accordingly.

If we are to believe legend, werewolves draw their power from the moon. The sight of a silvery moon peaking in the sky through wispy clouds sends them into a howling frenzy and they too charge off to cause havoc. So take care and stay indoors at the time. Our emotions are similarly erratic, fluctuating at different times of the month. The moon governs our instincts and feelings. Its position in our birth chart makes us responsive and over-sensitive at times or cold and indifferent.

Physically the moon rules the stomach and breasts and controls the lymphatic system and the flow of other bodily fluids. A detrimental moon placement in our chart can make us moody, moldy and slightly mad. If it is present in a watery sign of the zodiac like Cancer, Scorpio or Pisces, or conjoins a larger planet, like Neptune, Pluto or Jupiter in your chart then it could be an indicator of a large person with issues.

Some astrologers suggest dieting according to the lunar phases. This is based on the traditional moon calendar which outlines planting cycles and advises the best time for sowing crops, fertilizing and reaping for the best harvest. Your body too can be honed by the moon.

If you wish to begin a diet apparently you should do so at the time of the waning moon, just after the full moon, for best results. In this phase the body can apparently 'get rid of Scoriae poison and water' more easily. I have no idea what Scoriae is but it sounds nasty. It's either something bad you picked up off your Scorpio lover or a curvature of the spine. Either way you need to get rid of it. Fast.

During the waxing moon when the moon is becoming fuller you must be careful not to eat too many thickeners, like sweets or fats, which will lead to you getting fatter too. Furthermore at this time you mustn't eat too late in the day in case you wake up the next day wider than usual. On fruit days, which coincide with the moon in the fire signs of Aries, Leo, or Sagittarius, stick to beans, peas, eggplants and rice.

Please don't ask me to explain why because I'm not the scientific type. I'm still trying to get my head around gravity. The equation has me baffled. 'Your weight is a measure of the pull of gravity between you and the body you are standing on.' I don't think it would make any difference who I was standing on but if I had a choice I would opt for Brad Pitt. Still I don't know how he'd influence my weight. My libido yes, my hormones absolutely, but not my weight.

This statement is tricky too. 'If you double your mass, gravity pulls at you twice as hard.' Does this mean the heavier you are the more God is trying to eject you off the planet? Or that we're grappling twice as hard as anyone else not to fall off or that you're carrying the weight of the world on your shoulders? Opting to take the easy way out, I suggest if you're really worried about your weight, invest in a piece of property on the moon. Your weight on the moon is only 17% of what it is on earth. So if you weigh 200 pounds here, you'll weigh only 33 pounds on the moon. What an incredible weight loss with a minimum of effort. Better still book your passage over and drifting among the stars on your rocket ship minus gravity your weight is a welcome zero!

Enough about the moon. What about ethereal Neptune or the god Poseidon to the Greeks? Neptune, the water god, came from a powerful clan, being the son of Saturn and brother to Jupiter and Pluto. Still he was a mover in his own right. Ruler of the ocean, Neptune could whip up the waves with his three pronged trident and call forth storms or if in a better mood he could calm the seas and offer up a few fish or squid.

Neptune is the outermost planet of the gas giants. It is azure blue in color, like the ocean, with a faint and fragmented ring system. A nebulous, other worldly planet, it is the ruler of the last sign of the zodiac and the one considered the most highly evolved, Pisces. This sign represents spirituality and ultimate enlightenment.

Neptune is the master of illusion and so persons born under his influence can have a wonderful rich imagination or conversely can become delusional and lost. Piscean people have trouble dealing with the real world and may wish to escape reality. Neptune rules music and that's why many errant rock stars reach out to alcohol and drugs, the ultimate enticing brew that fall under the illusory god's spell.

As Neptune takes approximately fourteen years to pass through an astrological sign, it influences a whole generation of people. It's also the reason why music changes through the decades, reflecting the mood of the times. I was born when Neptune was in Libra, when music was sweet and sassy. Venus had her day and song lyrics were obsessed with love. Love found, lost and cried over. Just the way she likes it.

In the sixties, Neptune passed through Scorpio and music became deep and introspective. It was a time of drugs, psychedelic trips and warped dreams and the shadowy, mysterious world of the psyche. With the onset of the 21st century Neptune entered Aquarius, the sign of technology. Music became rap and techno and no longer did one switch on a radio. Instead it was downloaded from a computer and iPods were plugged into people's heads like an antenna. Music became less a creation than an invention and it was lost to me and other old souls.

Neptune also rules the area of the paranormal which is an extension of its ethereal vibration. People who possess the gift of heightened senses and psychic ability are Neptune's children. Highly sensitive to astral influences they are open to other planes of existence and can tune into energies that most people are oblivious to.

At the time of my birth, Neptune was positioned in the sky exactly next to the sun. This joining of the sun's soul essence with Neptune's spirituality is considered the mark of a psychic or astrologer. The extreme sensitivity associated with this conjunction can work against you. Flickering lights, noise and other stimuli affect me adversely and loud discordant people or music make me crazy.

Now to prove a point, on a more profound level the joining of these two planets had an even greater effect. The ocean has incredible depth and Neptune holds many watery secrets. Mine didn't come out for many years. The fact is I was born with a large brain which caused a build up of fluid in my skull. Yes, there was too much fluid around my brain which eventually seeped into my spinal cord and damaged it.

The operation to relieve the pressure and release the fluid was a risky one and I could have ended up with a permanent shunt inside my body to drain away the excessive fluid or even worse paralyzed or dead. Putting my faith in astrology to the test, I scheduled the surgery on the exact day that Jupiter, the planet of good fortune, trined or formed a perfect triangle in the sky to Saturn, the planet of health. It was the optimum day for the best outcome.

Just as I predicted and hoped, the surgery went perfectly with no need for a shunt. I had staked my life on astrology such was my belief in its accuracy. When people asked what was wrong with me I replied, 'My brain was too big so they had to make my head bigger so that it would fit.' Most people looked perplexed by my reply even though it is true while others joked, 'You must be really clever to have such a big brain.' We're back to the faulty equation. Thinking too much had made my brain big just as eating too much makes your body fat.

While some folk might be tempted to call me fathead now that my skull has expanded to accommodate my big brain, I have the last laugh. 'Size does matter, stupid,' were the headlines of a newspaper article, splashed above a photo of Einstein's brain which was found to be larger than the average brain. What a relief! Obviously with my sizeable brain I was clever just like Einstein or else Piscean Einstein suffered from a waterlogged head just like me.

POTENT PLUTO

Pluto was first spied hovering in the cosmos in 1930. Its discovery coincided with the rise of Fascism and Stalinism in Europe, in the lead up to the Second World War and the end of the Great Depression. It followed the birth of modern psychoanalysis as Freud and Jung explored the depths of the unconscious. Let's face it ... most of us would have needed therapy with all that negativity going on.

Pluto has recently been demoted from its status as a planet but we astrologers know better. This is one heavenly body not to be trifled with. It may be relatively small and may not conform precisely to planetary specifications but it is still a powerful player in the heavens. It is composed primarily of rock and ice. HEAVY rock and ice.

Pluto was the Roman god of the underworld and was dubbed Hades by the Greeks. We all know that Hades is not a place we hope to visit or spend any quality time in, a hell of a place really, so it's best to keep out of this ruthless god's path. In some Asian cultures he is known as Yama, the Guardian of Hell. Pluto is also considered the god of wealth because most of the world's riches are found beneath the earth's surface. Gold, oil, gas and a vast array of precious gems.

Pluto has his purpose because he challenges man to grow. He will scourge your soul until you catch a glimpse of the reserves that lie below the surface and is powerful enough to create pure crystal light out of the hardest granite soul. He takes little pleasure in superficial delights or in outward appearance. Pluto is much more concerned with depth and vision and if you haven't got any, watch out!

With an orbit that takes 248 years to complete, Pluto spends about twenty one years in each astrological sign. If Pluto touches on a sensitive spot in your chart ... ouch, you will be sorely tested. You will be a better person for the experience but it will still hurt. Little of consequence is gained easily so resign yourself to the pain and go beyond. Who knows what treasures you will uncover along the way?

People who were born when Pluto was joined to a personal planet in the sky are a touch above the rest. They possess an incredible amount of power and endurance and may have gone through agonizing times in past lives and are still bearing the scars. They can be wounded souls and the hurt may manifest it in a variety of ways, either destructive or transforming. They may also have been in an elevated position of power and now can use this power wisely or to manipulate and control.

Theories are bandied about that big people have been hurt or abused in the past and how their fat acts as a protective layer. Sorry, I don't agree. Most of the abused children I saw while counseling were gaunt and distressed and the only chubby child referred to me was a bit of a trickster, always craving fun and making trouble. Not to say that abuse does not present in all sizes and all forms but fat is not the determining factor.

People who are in pain, be it emotional, physical or psychic, can abuse substances to ease their angst but to say food is their drug of choice is misleading. Food is life giving, unlike alcohol and drugs or self mutilation or total withdrawal. We may reach out to food because it is comforting and basically tastes good. It makes us feel better but in a positive way. Overindulgence may be a cry for help but is more often a groan of frustration, for the deprivation we have been forced into.

It makes much more sense karmically that people who crave food in this lifetime to the point of overeating and creating an unhealthy fat buffer were deprived of food in the past. Think of the tens of millions of people who have died from starvation, pestilence, disease, drought, war and famine. It's logical that food for them would represent life and survival. It's the ultimate affirmation of life and all its bounty.

My parents endured dreadful experiences in World War 2. They were ripped away from their homelands at a young age, witnessed the loss of everything meaningful in their lives and were totally crushed when their families were put to death in front of their eyes.

My mother survived Auschwitz concentration camp by an act of God. She was sixteen at the time and had given up not only on life but also on God for allowing such atrocities to take place. In the end she was thin, frail and emaciated and became so ill that she had to be held up by the other women in the block at roll call so that she would not be put to death.

It was only after a German officer picked her to work in the kitchen that fate took a turn and she survived. She stayed alive by eating potato peelings, scraps that we regularly discard without a thought, saved her life. At night she looked through a small window, horrified and helpless, as the acrid smoke of people being burnt in the collective ovens blazed through the air. It was the Plutonic stench of death at its worst and she still suffers disturbing memories of it till today.

After his ordeal in Auschwitz, my father was sent to dismantle the infamous Warsaw ghetto. There he endured daily humiliation and beatings and woke each morning to be surrounded by corpses of men riddled with typhoid and starvation. They had given up the fight but my father was one of a steely handful who survived. Still the horrid scenes of death stayed embedded in his psyche where they are stamped forever, just like the obscene blue numbers tattooed on his arm.

Growing up as a child, my family life was emotional as my parents grappled with the ghosts of their past. One thing that my father always insisted on was that the dining table should be overflowing with food at mealtimes. There could never be enough. Salad, bread, meat, vegetables, fruit and desserts. Finished off with chocolates and nuts. The reason is obvious. Food represented life. It meant sanity, survival and hope. The ripe robust colors and textures, the stunning taste and aromas. After the grey and black of annihilation and starvation, food was God's gift. It mirrored the best life had to offer, not the worst.

FOOD IS VALUABLE BECAUSE IT REPRESENTS LIFE.

As anyone who has been sick can vouch for, one of the worst side effects of illness is the lack of appetite and subsequent loss of energy. Not to be able to savor the abundance of the earth is devastating so why people choose to do that voluntarily is inconceivable. If fat is trauma related and has resulted in the gaining of weight, diets will be counterproductive. These people equate loss of flesh as a lead up to eventual starvation and death. As soon as the message is relayed to the mind, the damaged psyche kicks in to protect the wounded soul. That wounded person will gorge themselves as a survival instinct and return to a weight with which they feel comfortable and safe.

The first three letters of diet spell DIE. People who are ill with AIDS, cancer and other devastating diseases literally waste away until they become a shadow of their former self. They will fight for survival at all costs and to them soft glowing flesh is a welcome sign of life. They crave to become whole once more and return to a wonderful state of health. It's all about living an abundant true life and being whole.

THE SKINNY PLANETS

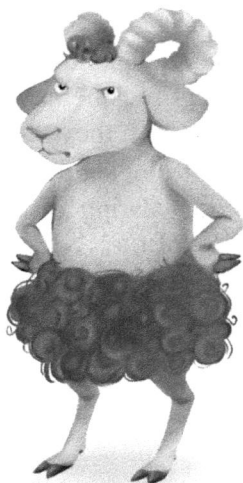

Now that we aware of the gifts and challenges handed down to us through the more abundant planets, let us look to the leaner signs of the zodiac. Generally these are the air and fire signs because they are the active, unstable elements. They feed off each other, fire and air. Fire sparks and burns brightly while air puffs and blows. Together they are explosive and fuel each other's energy to create and learn.

Both air and fire can rarely be contained unlike the other two elements, the more stable earth and water. These two can be collected, stored and remain constant. They can also be mixed together to make mud which explains why many of these signs are tedious 'stick in the muds'. It's pretty easy to guess what elements the singer Muddy Waters was born under, while the group Earth, Wind and Fire were unsure.

Let's begin with the most dramatic of all, fire. Fire is volatile and spreads quickly until it rages out of control. The Fire signs are Aries, Leo and Sagittarius. Fire people burn up a lot of energy so those born under these signs usually have a strong metabolism, fuelled by a mighty furnace. They are so active they care little for food or else gulp it down with such little thought they scarcely have time to digest it. They are naturally slim signs, so piling on weight is rarely an issue.

The first of the fire signs, Aries, is powered by Mars, the god of war and rampant destruction. With energy and anger to burn, it's best not to cross him or get in his way. Always on the march in search of a new foe or for a village to burn, Aries is usually lean or muscular. He furrows his brow and glares a lot, so Arians are usually identifiable by their distinctive eyebrows, like the horns of their animal sign the Ram.

Aries celebrities of the raised brow and slender frame include Adrien Brody, Jennifer Garner and Keira Knightly. The anger of Mars manifests in the temper of feisty Russell Crowe, Shannon Doherty and Diana Ross. Rams love to kick and fight like Jackie Chan and Lucy Lawless as Xena, the Warrior Princess, while Aries directors show their violent side in film. Quentin Tarantino with Kill Bill and Pulp Fiction, and Francis Ford Coppola in Apocalypse Now. The real deal was Adolf Hitler, just edging out of Aries and hovering on the brink of Taurus, and you couldn't get any darker or more destructive than him.

Leo, the lion, is the second of the fire signs. Leos range from purring pussycats to roaring tigers, with delicious catlike features. These can manifest in the feline eyes of Madonna, Kim Cattrell, and Sandra Bullock, the thick mane of hair of Debra Messing, or the aristocratic bearing of Charlize Theron and Helen Mirren. Some rangy tom cats include Billy Bob Thornton and Mick Jagger, while Leo Lisa Kudrow's favorite song on Friends was Smelly Cat.

With Sagittarius, the last of the fire signs, it's all about the legs. Ruled by Jupiter, it is the archer, half man and half horse. Horses have stout flanks and strong legs and love to gallop. As do those born under this sign. A great example is the 1940's pin up girl Betty Grable, whose fabulous legs were insured by her Hollywood studio for one million dollars each with Lloyds of London! Daryl Hannah transformed her long legs into a mermaid tail, while Jane Fonda made a fortune bouncing around on hers and Lucy Lui kicked her way to fame in Charlie's Angels. Then there are leggy Teri Hatcher and Kim Basinger and who could forget Brad Pitt's bronzed thighs in Troy.

Now let's take a look at the air signs. The intellectuals of the zodiac, they are more inclined towards high brow pursuits. They utilize energy through their minds, which streamlines their bodies. Geminis and Aquarians would prefer to read a book or sit at their computer rather than eat. Food for them is less of a comfort than a necessity.

Geminis, ruled by the planet Mercury, are usually tall and agile. The sign of the twins, they burn enough energy for two and can hardly sit still before darting off on another project. They suffer with restless leg syndrome where their body tries to keep up with their mind. They're people on the move, with lots to do. A case in point is Angelina Jolie who seems to possess superhuman energy as she raises a brood of children, shoots another movie and then jets off to save the world. Other Geminis are the enigmatic and lean Nicole Kidman, Annette Benning and Johnny Depp.

The air sign of Aquarius is ruled by the unstable planet Uranus. It governs electricity, lightning and anything powered by an energy source. Aquarians do not have much of an appetite and have probably beamed down from another planet and some could be aliens in disguise. Elfin and gamin, they appear in the guise of the slim and petite actresses Mia Farrow, Christina Ricci, Jennifer Aniston, Ellen DeGeneres and Portia de Rossi.

The air sign Libra is the exception to the slender air rule. Granted they are a bright lot with more than their fair share of intelligence but with Venus as their nubile ruler, Librans would prefer to spend time at the beauty salon having a relaxing facial or massage. That's a true test of their IQ because they've gotten their priorities right. They also like to read, preferably while eating a bowl of strawberries dipped in chocolate.

Now for a completely different perspective let's swing over to the ancient land of India to get an Eastern slant on the subject of weight. The traditional health practice of Ayurveda has been handed down over centuries in the subcontinent and incorporates holistic and natural methods for optimum health. In its wisdom it recognizes three main body types, each with different dispositions and body shapes.

I definitely belong to the Kapha type who are described as easygoing, relaxed, affectionate, forgiving, compassionate and loving. Physically they are strong types with a sturdy, heavier build. Yet despite their bulk they are graceful and slow to anger. Their hair and skin is soft and lustrous and they have large eyes and a mellow voice. They also attract wealth and are reportedly enduring in bed.

I'm liking this list. People with a kapha constitution have well developed bodies, with broad chests and big breasts. Now here comes the rub, there had to be one. Kapha people have regular appetites but due to their sluggish digestion they usually *eat less food but put on weight*. However some good news, despite these undeserved extra pounds they sleep soundly and are healthy and peaceful people.

On the negative side, Kapha folk are prone to heavy, oppressive depressions. This is especially the case if they move to the West where they fail to be appreciated. Who wouldn't be depressed when you're being so badly discriminated against? Being the non-judgmental and tolerant sorts, Kaphas will forgive you and move on which tends to be their undoing because it lets the rest get away with murder, at least of the spirit. However there is karma to be had here.

It seems the other two groups don't fare so well. The Pitta type comes off reasonably OK. They are of medium physique and have a sharp focused mind. They have a strong appetite naturally and *can digest large quantities of food and liquids and get away with it*. However with their stubborn headstrong attitude they can become easily irritated and angry. With their speedy metabolism what have they got to be so peeved about? No wonder our lot has to be forgiving. Pitta types sound like fire signs gone wild but an inferno by any other name is still an inferno, no matter what continent you're on.

The third type, Vatas, are a bit of a worry. They are described as physically undeveloped with flat chests and protruding veins and tendons. In LA they can pump up a flat chest but it's hard to strip a protruding vein or unfurl a bothersome tendon. Vatas are the anxious type and their skin is cold and rough, at worst dry and cracked. Their 'hair is scant, eyelashes are thin and their eyes are listless and their noses bent.' You wouldn't want to bump into a drunken Vata in a dark alley late at night or be introduced to one on a blind date.

Indians are into astrology so you don't have to look too closely to see the planetary correlations on their list. Luscious Venus bestowing her charms on all those plump Kaphas with her gorgeous lush locks, radiant smile and loving ways. Mars is raging on the side of the Pittas, who sweat a lot because of all that blocked energy. Pittas are strangely described as blond or redhead, which bodes the question of where are we exactly in India? Do I sense a lingering hostility against the British colonialists?

As for those scrawny Vatas, blame Mercury and Uranus for your lot. The only advice I can offer is to pack your bags and head straight to Hollywood. Invest in a skilled personal trainer and a top plastic surgeon, get some silicone boobs and a nose job and you're set. For the boys, a firm butt implant wouldn't go astray. As for me, I'm heading for Mumbai for a good veggie curry and a buttered naan.

WHAT SECRET?

I'm all for the power of positive thinking but I'm also a realist. A healthy dose of cynicism tempers my Neptunian idealism to help me better cope with an imperfect world, with all its inherent lessons. As an astrologer I'm also well aware of the higher truths that govern the affairs of man. Whatever our hopes and dreams may be, we cannot determine the conditions of our passage or guarantee its outcome.

To simplify our existence by reducing it to the laws of attraction, or to believe that if you wish for something hard enough then it will become yours, is naïve. There is much more to the process than getting what you want out of life. If we all had a genie in a bottle and could wish our way through life, would we really be happy? True wealth often comes from that which is not easily gained, for it is only through the effort that we come to appreciate what is truly valuable.

Let's face it. If we could all wish ourselves slim, there would be few fat people left on the earth. Not because we devalue who we are but because we have been *taught* to value ourselves less. Imagine if we were all slim. What a wonderful world it would be, full of shiny, happy people! The appeal of living in Pleasantville wears thin after a while and to aspire to have a million dollars or a mansion in the Hollywood hills or to be a 'perfect' shape is vacuous and lacking in worth. Is that the best we can hope for? What about understanding and wisdom?

The universe is not as shallow as we pretend to be nor is there a fairy godmother handing out gifts to make our passage effortless. There are lessons to be learned. That's the reason we're here. These lessons might come to you unexpectedly. That gold necklace you yearn for in the shop window may be the reason you get mugged on your Brazilian holiday and the bright red convertible might just up end up killing you.

Bad things happen. We cannot wish them away nor should we. It's a sobering fact that real depth of soul is created out of the pulp of life. From the events we are sometimes forced to endure and the people and circumstances that have challenged us to grow in the most excruciating, painful, introspective and soul curdling way. Good times are just the icing on the cake, the pot of gold at the end of the rainbow.

Depth is a Saturn thing. Saturn takes about twenty eight years to complete one cycle, and it puts you through the wringer so that you might learn and grow. The four angles of Saturn represent the major turning points in our development. At seven we leave behind our childhood fantasies, at fourteen we reach puberty, at twenty one we are given the key to the door and at twenty eight we reach adulthood. When Saturn returns to its starting position in your horoscope, that's when everything falls into place for you have completed a crucial cycle.

The end of the first Saturn cycle marks the primary consolidation of self. Ready to assume more responsibility people marry, change jobs or residences and make other important life changes. Unfortunately they can also die. It appears they have come into this incarnation for one time round, to learn something specific. With their task complete it's time to leave. It's hard to accept and even harder to comprehend.

The death of the talented actor Heath Ledger at twenty eight is a recent example. Kurt Cobain, the lead singer of Oasis, died at twenty seven from a self inflicted gunshot to the head and Jim Morrison of the Doors died at the same age of a drug overdose. At twenty eight Brandon Lee died when shot from a dummy pistol on set, Janis Joplin passed from a drug overdose and Jimi Hendrix died from a mixture of wine and sleeping pills. One chance to shine brightly and then fade out, but as legendary icons their memory remains with us forever.

With the passing of such major talent we can take comfort in the fact that death is less a tragedy and more an awakening. I believe in the concept of reincarnation as do most Hindus and Buddhists. As such, death is not final but rather just part of the eternal wheel of life.

Saturn's second cycle is completed around fifty six years of age, its third at approximately eighty four. Check the obituaries. At these ages many people pass over. That is not to say that people don't die at other times, which obviously they do, but a great number follow the Saturnian path and bow out at the end of a specific learning phase.

While we're talking learning, let's take a look at the dark broody planet of Pluto. It takes many years to move and if it challenges a crucial point in your birth chart you will be sorely tested. As hard as it is to accept, you chose to undergo this trial before you got here or it was thrust upon you because there is something you needed to learn or there was some karmic imbalance that had to be addressed or righted.

No amount of wishing or hoping will stop the process for it is one of the main reasons you are here. To learn, process and grow. Pluto allows you time to work through a previous injustice or to right a wrong and time to assimilate it. Through the ordeal you must let go of the residue of the past so the soul is free to continue on its journey.

You don't need an astrologer to tell you when Pluto is overhead, you will know. A dark cloud will descend upon you to extinguish your light. Take heart for you will emerge a better person for it. You will survive to emerge from your hour of darkness, transformed.

Now back to the power of positive thinking. When it was all the rage I stuck inspirational sayings on my freezer hoping to transform my thinking and stop myself from opening the refrigerator door. Happy thoughts like, 'I'm trim and terrific.' 'I'm in a wonderful relationship.' 'I'm healthy and content.' 'My home is a peaceful retreat.'

I repeated the words dutifully every day but all my efforts to create a wondrous reality failed miserably. I never transformed into a beauteous swan, my partner turned out to be an unstable schizophrenic and I hovered on death's doorstep due to a serious medical condition that went undetected for years. Recovering from surgery, I was barraged with noise as the flight path shifted right over my apartment.

Did I wish this on myself? No way. It was my worst nightmare and I couldn't even begin to imagine such an abysmal reality let alone create it. Was I bad at affirmations, not really believing they were going to work? Well, I did my best. I tried to believe. Or was it that my expectations were unreasonable or that I deserved to suffer?

None of the above. The truth was that I was already a swan but I couldn't see it, having been quashed by a society that concentrates on one's perceived shortcomings rather than celebrates the essence of one's beauty. As for my relationship, the trials with my partner taught me to be compassionate but also how to establish boundaries. After years of pain, my illness was finally diagnosed and the surgery saved my life, adding fuel to my belief that every moment of life is precious and is to be enjoyed to the max. As for the airplanes flying over my head, I have yet to decipher the meaning of such an aerial assault except to serve as a not so subtle reminder that I need to be living elsewhere.

While I was going through these trials I was miserable but I had every right to be. To be sad in difficult situations is both comforting and healing. If I was running down the hills singing in ecstasy dodging all manner of missiles, like a Swiss milk maid yodeling across the Swiss Alps at the height of a bomber attack, or sliding down the mountainside gleefully on a block of Toblerone, would I be nuts or not?

Absolutely. To be in a constant state of euphoria, no matter what hand life deals you, is absurd. Don't get me wrong. Positive thinking has a part to play. When you use it well, to contemplate what you would like to attract into your life and be ready when the time is right, when the universe offers it up to you, that's intelligent and optimal. It's best served when you use it to draw on your reserves. To find the strength and resolve to crush the beast, no matter what that beast may be.

My ethereal friend Ingrid is always full of positive vibes and sound advice. She inspires me to think good thoughts and eat muesli each morning to stay regular. However when she suggested after a painful break-up with a cruel partner that I should forgive him and send him off in a bubble of love and light, I was incensed. I wanted to tie him to a stake in the middle of a snowfield and fire a cannon!

I cannot wish him well. At least not yet. I am licking my wounds and he has wounded me. Deeply. It will take a long time to heal and slowly my anger will dissipate and become a long forgotten friend, to be replaced by acceptance and an uneasy peace. Maybe one day I can smile when I see him again. Perhaps I will even be able to forgive him. But feelings are valid, valuable and not easily manipulated. Instead they should be honored.

Now I'm not averse to having conversations with God. I often do. I ask for the occasional sign, nothing too showy or demanding like the parting of the Red Sea but a warm fuzzy moment to remind me of his presence. I have asked for his help at times of need and spoken to him about my hopes and dreams. I'm not alone in my great aspirations.

One of my favorite scenes in a movie is when Bette Midler played the author Jacqueline Sussan who wrote the book 'Valley of the Dolls'. Miss Sussan apparently had long talks with the Almighty in the park, begging him to let her rise above her mediocrity as a two bit actress and to be famous one day. She was a Leo, so she couldn't help herself. However God did not grant her wish, at least not at first.

Instead she went through times of tragedy after giving birth to an autistic son who was institutionalized for most of his life, and then had some more bad breaks before she learnt she had breast cancer. That was it! Storming into the park, incensed by the injustice of it all, she shouts at God while her husband tries to restrain her. 'Damn you!' she flares. 'All I wanted was to be famous, couldn't you at least do that.'

Eventually God relented and Valley of the Dolls became one of the best selling books of all time, selling more than thirty million copies. It went on to become a film sensation so she got her wish in the end. I'm still waiting for mine but it's all a matter of good luck and timing, which my publisher reminds me of constantly. If we all got our wish there would be no more heartbroken writers with enough rejection slips to wallpaper their homes. Not to mention all the other bruised creative hearts who miss out on their dream.

Miss Sussan got her wish but she didn't have long to appreciate it. She died of breast cancer at the age of fifty six, at the end of her second Saturn cycle. Others who passed at this time include Beethoven who died of lead poisoning, the singers George Harrison, Bill Haley, Bob Marley, Dan Fogelberg, Ian Drury, Luther Vandross, Roger Miller, John Entwistle, Tammy Wynette, Robin Gibb, Rick James, Barry White, Del Shannon from a self inflicted gun shot wound, Linda McCartney, the horror actor Bela Lugosi, the James Bond author Ian Fleming and the world's oldest pony Sugar Puff who died at fifty six.

See, 'sugar' does apparently make you live longer! There's a saying, 'be careful what you wish for because you might just end up getting it.' Things are not always as they seem. One night I was at the local club feeling somewhat dejected. I took refuge in the poker machines because I like to watch the colored wheels spin. I'm not a serious gambler not like some freewheeling Jupitereans who don't know when to stop. That particular night I was disappointed.

There were no bells or flashing lights and no winning streak. Nothing to cheer me up. To add to my misery when I took my handbag off the ledge, I noticed it had been moved. Then to my horror I realized my wallet had been stolen, along with all my cash and credit cards. I started to panic. It was Friday night and the banks were closed for the weekend. How could I have been so stupid, so careless? I hadn't been vigilant enough. What sort of sick joke was the cosmos playing on me? I had asked for the best and had gotten the worst.

With tears welling up, I was shown to the manager's office. After cancelling my credit cards over a cup of tea and slice of apple pie, I was escorted to the police station. After reporting the crime I went back to the club. The manager insisted I eat dinner and was shown to the a la carte restaurant to order whatever I wanted. I was too upset to eat but then I thought what the heck! I'd never had such an offer before so I decided to eat my way through the menu. King prawns for appetizer, fruit cocktails, roast duck with fresh figs followed by yummy crepe suzette for dessert. I felt like I'd gone to Heaven. My tears dried up.

Then when I was about to leave the club the manager came over and insisted that I come to the club any time over the weekend and eat whatever I wanted. He then instructed the club driver to take me home and escort me to the door, before handing me an envelope that contained $100. 'It's from me,' he said, 'just pay it back when you can.' I was overwhelmed by his kindness. The following week, I was invited back to the club for dinner to be informed of the steps they had taken to locate the thief, who they had captured perfectly on camera.

Now, every time I go to the club the staff are incredibly nice and always say hello. The manager has become a friend and often invites me to join him for a chat and a drink. What a wonderful blessing that was given to me, far superior to the trivial one I asked for. Last time I enquired the thief was in prison after committing some other offence so he got what he deserved and definitely *not* what he wished for.

I learnt so much from that experience. Sometimes we are short-sighted not recognizing tough circumstances are blessings in disguise, the proverbial silver lining in a dark sky brimming with storm clouds. There is much more to our passage than riches and material wealth or the superficiality of outer appearance. If you were offered the choice between looking like a Hollywood celebrity and being yourself, I think you would be surprised with the answer. We only think we want to be different. In truth we just want to be our personal best. OUR BEST.

We should strive towards being our optimum self and progress towards the evolution of our soul because that is the reason we were put on this planet in the first place. So grab life's opportunities, whatever form they come to you in, and rise to the occasion. At the end of the day you will be proud of who you are. The person who you were meant to be. Look into the mirror of the universe and *see* yourself, then smile. Say I LOVE YOU, to every adorable inch of you whether it is lumpy, bumpy or lean!

LET THE BRAINWASH BEGIN

Weight is a billion dollar business and a fortune is spent trying to shed unwanted pounds and rid ourselves of assorted bulges that we are not fond of, or at least tighten them up or smooth them down a bit. In the process we make ourselves miserable. Our society has led the way, degrading us even more. As I flicked through a new edition of a popular Woman's magazine this is what I found.

A real teaser. A bra ad with a beautiful plus size model, so we're doing well. Unfortunately the by-line is not so encouraging. 'Nothing should get in the way of looking fabulous' Do they mean our breasts? 'So if you agree that less really is more try it for yourself and feel great.' I wish it was that easy. Now, I have no objection to trying to curb your curves if your breasts stick out like giant bazookas in your sweater but I'm not convinced that more really is less.

This ad is followed by a sad story about actress Kirstie Alley and her path to ruination with bloated pictures of her devouring a box of fried chicken in a variety of unflattering poses. Once again she is out of control they claim and has let her weight slide out from under her. Slim by nature, Kirstie's overeating well may be a sign of a deeper problem but having unseemly photos of her in the glossies is not the answer.

Skipping over the next few pages of the magazine we come to the cookery section packed with lots of temptations. This week it's, 'Sweet Treats. Popular indulgences that have stood the test of time.' With mouth watering photos of White Chocolate Napoleon Cake, Rainbow Layer Cake and Passionfruit Melting Moments among others. Yum!

A few pages further on we have a full page ad with some poor wretch grappling to do up the zipper of her jeans. 'Hate feeling like a before photo?' The lass has obviously been indulging in some of the sweets on the previous page or has merely bought the wrong size jeans and is now paying the price. Perhaps in the future dessert recipes should be presented in a sealed section, classified, 'For thin eyes only.'

Then comes a swish ad claiming a famous swimming star has lost forty pounds in just a few months by drinking a brand of diet shake. In fact 20% of his body weight. He felt depressed and worthless before, when he was flab instead of fab. Not only is he now transformed but along the way he stumbled on the diet industry's ***dirty little secret.*** According to the blurb, it seems many diet shakes contain a shocking amount of sugar! Am I surprised? Do I care? Will it stop the earth turning or result in global warming? I think not. In any case I tried a diet shake once but couldn't stomach it so I ate a donut instead.

Several pages on there is a full page ad with a rather disturbing headline. 'How to turn your body into An Automatic Fat Burner'. I have terrible visions of self combustion and a pile of ashes lying on the floor where a person used to be! In truth I'd rather turn my body into an Automatic Oil Burner and have lavender essence exude from every pore so I won't have to ever buy deodorant again!

Anyway the ad makes this incredible claim. 'Imagine eating six meals a day and in less than 30 days you will be able to look at yourself in the mirror and hardly recognize the person staring back at you.' Scary stuff. Would I see Freddy Kruger, Florence Henderson of the Brady Bunch, or Marlon Brando at his worst staring back at me? Or a silhouette paper cut out of the real me. Really, really scary stuff. Why make the insinuation that you want to see anyone other than yourself?

Then comes the best of all. A full length article titled, 'How to Get Healthy at Home. Nifty tricks for helping you beat the battle of the bulge.' Color is the key here. According to research, red, yellow and orange are colors that stimulate the appetite and are thus used by the fast food companies to entice you to enter their golden arches. The food tastes pretty good too which is an even greater incentive.

Blue on the other hand is a color that rarely occurs in nature, which begs the question, 'what about the sky and sea?' which are forever expansive and all around us. The writer states there are no blue vegetables or meat, unless they're off. So what about blueberries, blackcurrants, blackberries, boysenberries and rainbow ice-cream? Blue suppresses the appetite so if you're serious about losing weight paint your kitchen blue, buy blue serviettes and dinner plates because it will put you off your food. Strange because Wedgwood did OK with its blue willow pattern but maybe it's left on the dresser just for show.

Once you've got your colors sorted out, confront your bulk by putting a mirror near places where you tend to eat. Shriek! I don't want to see myself doing the dirty deed, that's worse than watching my boobs flop during sex. I want to enjoy both acts. It's bad enough that I have to look in a mirror to brush my teeth but otherwise I avoid them like the plague. Now I'm supposed to stare at myself stuffing an oozing cream cake into my mouth or crunching on a chicken bone.

I'd rather eat glass and in a fit of Greek pique may just smash all the mirrors in my house. If the sound of shattering glass doesn't appeal, move your CD player into the kitchen. Music influences the 'pleasure systems' in our brain it states and the faster the beat the more we tend to eat. So if you want to pile on weight then play 'Flight of the Bumblebee'. To lose pounds it seems flute music works the best. I think a funeral march would have more impact or even better the rap version of 'I like big butts and cannot lie', or 'Who let the dogs out?'

After hiding the remote so you can't indulge in mindless eating while watching TV, go round the house and change all the lights bulbs. It's best if the rooms where you eat have bright glaring light to make you more self conscious. Might I suggest a spotlight as a good investment or a large mirror ball in the living room so you can dance under it to remind yourself of good times when you didn't give a toss.

So to sum up if you want to lose weight, paint your kitchen blue, set the table with a winsome bluebird design and sing 'Am I Blue?' or 'Blue Bayou' as a sign of your depression, to the accompaniment of Flutes of the Andes. Paste mirrors on the ceiling and walls, light the room with neons and then sit down to dinner. As a final touch I suggest you do all of the above in the nude because that will really put you off your food. In fact you may never, ever want to eat again!

The mixed messages we receive are not restricted to magazines. I love my morning shows on television and am very impressed that an assortment of ladies feature on the panels, proving that sharp wit and intelligence comes in all shapes and sizes. Large ladies on these shows are just as attractive as the rest and in some cases a lot more appealing. Talk show hosts and news announcers are often the standard package perhaps fuelled by network bosses who think we only want to watch the 'cream' of our species, a popular myth that needs to be shattered.

The most successful of them all, Oprah, did not reach the heights of success merely for her sharp insights. She did so also because she is an attractive larger woman who many of us can relate to. Ratings did not plummet when she gained weight but rather eased off when she was at her leanest and became obsessed with physical issues like diet and exercise. What a waste when there are so many more interesting topics to capture our interest. We prefer her curvaceous and glowing with life and enthusiasm rather than slim, self deprecating and full of doubt.

Real confusion sets in when live shows have the inevitable enticing cookery segment, full of delights to tempt the palate and rumble the stomach, followed by a string of ads to burn off fat, flatten your stomach and tone up your abs. If we are to believe the hype that we have to twirl ourselves into oblivion for hours or climb Mt Everest to burn off a single cookie, then why bother? To add to the gloom is the funeral cover ad just in case you don't succeed or are thrust out of your bedroom window on your twirler, or another such tortuous exercise device, and land on your head.

When we are ordered to banish our 'love handles that nobody loves' our spirit is deflated if not our stomachs. Look at the term. Love handle. Something loving to hold on to in the height of passion or when you're having a stroll in the park and clinging onto the love of your life. There is something reassuring about soft and cuddly, as ads for fabric softeners happily remind us. When my lover honed his abs until they were rock hard I was put off. He was gorgeous in any case but it felt like I had a metal robot for a lover. I begged him to keep some of his moist flesh so I had something soft to hold onto and luckily he did.

If the images we see in ads are any indicators, with their string of perfect slender people, then normal or chubby people don't wash their hair or use beauty products, (even though they most often have radiant skin and lustrous hair) or never get cold sores, acne or have a headache. They also don't buy cars, cleaning fluids or household products. Ironically they also don't appear to eat or drink which is strange considering they've been accused of eating too much. So it appears that no one wants their product associated with a 'normal' or plus size person even though they might be their target market. Shame on you.

The only current ads on TV using larger persons are demeaning, a caricature of a woman with a matching rotund bulldog and some floozy dame stuffing her mouth with donuts for some car business I want nothing to do with. While it may be 'lovely' to see a lean lass splashing perfume on her body while running under the Eiffel Tower thinking ethereal thoughts, like where she can purge on the Left Bank before the next shot or how appetizing her celery stick will be for lunch, it is not inspiring. It does not inspire me to buy the product nor does it make me aspire to be like her one day. It's never going to happen.

Start to show a range of normal, attractive people in ads so that we can relate to them, like Dove did with their beauty products. When cosmetic companies use a top model with perfect skin to convince us that their moisturizer is best, I don't buy it. They were perfect before so where's the improvement? Show me someone like myself, glowing with life and happiness after using it and then you've got a sale.

When major department stores use a world class beauty as their spokesperson, one who was voted the most stunning in the universe either in a beauty contest or in the modeling world, they set an impossible standard. While no doubt they're attractive to look at, they are unreachable and unattainable. Not only would I not rush out to buy the dress they're wearing but I couldn't even get it over my head or yank my wrist through the sleeve. It's time we lived in the real world.

By all means keep the so called 'best' but add the rest. Show us women we can relate to, wearing clothes we can wear. Encourage designers to add larger sizes to their collections so that we can actually fit into them and then add more designers who know their stuff and can design fabulous outfits to flatter all shapes at an affordable price. This is a true measure of beauty, one that is way overdue. Make us feel prized, special and beautiful rather than making us feel that we don't measure up. Just take a look at the women sitting in the audience of these television shows. All shapes, all backgrounds, all types. Most feeling less than they should be instead of the best that they can be, and that's the greatest tragedy of all. It's time for a major shift in consciousness.

DIET OR DIE

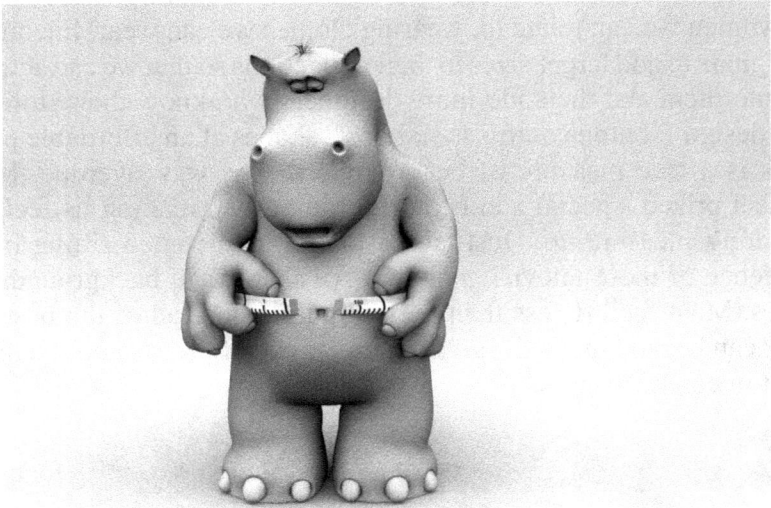

An anagram of diet is 'edit'. Edit means to cut down or to amend the original version. Then there's 'tied' because when you diet you're bound to some ridiculous regime that you resent. Diet also can be spelt from the word deprivation which is not natural to the human condition. People resort to extreme measures to lose weight and very few with permanent or satisfying results. It was recently reported that 95% of people who lose a substantial amount of weight will put it back on within a year. That's a whole lot of effort just to feel frustrated and fail.

It's not that we're all terrible dieters but rather that we don't *want* to diet. Most normal people don't want to deny themselves and even worse concentrate on food and calories all the time. We just want to get on with life and enjoy what we love the most. As a result weight will creep back on after dieting till it reaches *our* 'normal' level.

When a person has to resort to drastic procedures like stomach stapling and gastric banding then something is inherently wrong.

While these methods may be justified in cases where morbid obesity is life threatening, the whole concept is unnatural. If a person's stomach needs to be reduced in capacity so that it can only hold a thimble full of food, doesn't that imply by its very nature that it's abnormal? The ordinary person would starve in such a situation so the obese person obviously has very little capacity to burn off food or metabolize it.

Singer Carnie Wilson, who has faced an ongoing battle with her weight, gained over forty pounds even though she underwent gastric bypass in 1999. The body has a remarkable capacity, despite anything that has been done to it, to return to its natural state whatever that may be. That's why diets don't work. As I said before, you can't change species. With extreme measures one may initially lose weight but gradually it will pile back on until you make a life style change that you approve of and that suits your natural state of being.

A TV program recently showed a couple in their mid fifties who were practicing a severe form of food restriction in a bid to prolong their lives. In the future one could live to be one hundred and forty the program asserted, and this couple were well on their way to that goal by eating only twice a day, breakfast and lunch. Their meager meals consisted of only a handful of grains and vegetables. It reminds me of the strange theory that man can live by only breathing in the life giving rays of the sun and not eating at all. Unless you're an impoverished Indian swami on a massive head trip, why on earth would you bother?

Once again here's the crucial question. Why prolong life if you don't enjoy it? The deprived couple looked gaunt and uninspired, as do many strict food disciplinarians who seem grey and old before their time. It's not enough just to exist. You have to be ALIVE. Some of the medics and health gurus leading the fight against obesity look thin, craggy and pale, not brimming with life and vitality as one would expect. They're a mix of Mars domination, wanting everyone to buckle down, with Saturn's need to enforce and deny in the name of 'health'.

I would never aspire to look like these people because they lack the glow that comes from the joy of life. That spark is obtained by living an authentic life, living your passion whatever that may be. When I look back over my photos taken over the years, I was at my leanest when I was most depressed. I was going through turbulent times and the stress made me thin and gaunt. My happiest days were in the country where I enjoyed a great social life with lots of afternoon teas of scones and sponge cakes. I was chubby but happy, and extremely content.

American Dr. Robert Atkins devised the famous 'Atkins diet'. He advocated a high protein, low carbohydrate regime as the key to losing weight. I became ill on the diet as did others who could not handle the strict protein requirement. Dr. Atkins was a Libran like myself. As the sign of the scales, Libra is the only inanimate sign of the zodiac and is a pointed way to keep a check on Venus with her overindulgent ways.

Libra is also the sign of balance, prompting you to either swing wildly from eating binges to fasts until you find your center of balance. Balance proved literally to be Dr. Atkin's downfall because he died from complications after he slipped on the icy pavement outside his office. Simply, *he lost his balance.* Leaked death records maintained that he weighed 255 pounds at the time of his death. This was definitely not the lean figures expected of a diet guru. These claims were denied by his people who argued this weight gain was caused when his organs shut down. Whatever the cause it was the ultimate irony, illustrating that we rarely have control over anything, least of all our weight.

Statistics show that Mississippi is the fattest state in the USA, a country which has a total of 72 million overweight people. Here we have an example of poor diet which leads to dire consequences. The traditional diet of the south has taken its toll, with loads of fried foods cooked in pork fat and salt. Obviously this diet is an unhealthy one and needs to be drastically altered to improve the quality of life of people who suffer as a result. It's difficult to change eating habits but not impossible. It begins with education about healthy living and a vital acknowledgement that your body and spirit deserves the best. It's also about understanding that it's not quantity but quality that counts.

Dieting can be just as detrimental as overeating, especially when we put our body through the wringer and go from one extreme to the other. Many diets are not based on healthy premises but rather extreme measures which in turn will cause your body to go into shock and shed a few pounds which it will pile back on again at the first sign that the coast is clear and it can return to being normal. Consider this unhealthy batch of fad diets, designed either to whip you into shape or kill you.

The Cabbage Soup Diet sounds delectable as does the Hollywood Diet, a concoction of prune juice, assorted fruit juices, green tea and grape seed extract. Both are gas powered and will have you running to the nearest loo many times over and everyone else running to get out of your way! The Russian Air Force Diet is another winner. Day one consists of a cup of coffee for breakfast, two eggs and a tomato for lunch, and seven ounces of red meat and a green salad for dinner. I'd be wanting to stay out of Russian Air Space for safety reasons. One diet guaranteed to knock you off is the Lemonade Diet. NO food is allowed. Instead you ingest a mix of water, fresh lemon juice, maple syrup and cayenne pepper. In the morning you flush your body out with one quart of water and 2 teaspoons of salt, and at night a cup of Herbal Laxative Tea.

That diet is all set to blast the Russian pilots out of the sky and have everyone in tinsel town running for cover! Supermodel Naomi Campbell, among other celebrities, admits to guzzling a similar potent mix, sometimes for up to eighteen days at a time. The woman deserves to be slim. If it was me I would have keeled over from toxic poisoning and lack of interest within the first few hours. Mind you, if someone offered me zillions of dollars to walk down the catwalk showing off my newly honed but still chubby 5' 4' body I may just be tempted to give it a try.

The basic premise of the Blood Type diet advocated by Dr. Peter D'Adamo is that your blood type determines which food best suits you. Unfortunately most physicians, nutritionists and dieticians don't agree with him. Still if you're interested, here goes. Type O blood group is believed to be the hunter, the earliest human blood group. So the diet for this muscular, active group is one that is rich in meat. Chuck in a few veggies anyway, some plump carrots, corn and peas, so that you have a bit of color on your plate and on your cheeks.

The A blood group is the cultivator, dating back to the dawn of agriculture. So no red meat for this lot, rather a plate full of spinach, leeks and beans. If you get a chance, sneak behind the garden shed and devour a full bucket of fried chicken or at least munch on a tasty wing while pretending to dig a new veggie plot for the spring harvest.

Type B people are the nomads of the bunch. They have a strong immune system and a flexible digestive system and are apparently the only ones who can thrive on dairy products. Now I don't want to appear disbelieving but I'm type B. *B positive* to be precise which may just carry a hidden meaning. To disprove his point I'm lactose intolerant, however I have lived through plague and pestilence and love to move around from place to place so the doctor was right in some measure.

Blood group AB gets the best of both worlds, being a mixture of type A and B. So you lot get to throw both meat and vegetables on the plate and not feel guilty. Some guys have all the luck. I bet you're allowed dessert too. Last but not least is the Cardiologist's diet. Simple but true. 'If it tastes good, spit it out.' That just about sums it up.

After reading many articles about diets I was struck by one recurring theme. DIETS DON'T WORK, at least not in the long term for the majority of people. Typical is this woman's story, 'I have counted calories for decades, trying everything from the grapefruit diet to a regimen based on cabbage soup. I have also done Weight Watchers, twenty nine times. I knew it wouldn't be successful but I was desperate so I went back anyways.' Some would argue that she cheated or her attitude was self defeating, programming her for failure. I argue otherwise. As she goes on to say 'I thought I could be a size 10 but as it turned out I ended up roughly an 18 which is exactly where I started.'

Does anyone get it? The woman is meant to be a size 18 and her ideal weight matches a size 18, based on her family background, genetic and medical history and astrological inclination. What is wrong with being a size 18, after all? Who says size 10 is better than an 18? They're only numbers, just like our age which we also like to keep under wraps because it too is not a true indicator of how we feel or act. You can be healthy and attractive whatever your age or size, unless you're an extreme size zero in the shape of a starving supermodel, a traveler suffering from a diabolical gastric bug or some poor unfortunate dying of starvation in the middle of the Kalahari desert in Africa.

Size zero is OK if that is the size you were *meant* to be. If you are of Asian extraction or a lithe Aquarian or lean Aries or Capricorn it suits. For the rest of us it's a definite no. To be that size is unnatural for a person of a fuller build and will do more harm than good. Just as you cannot grow taller like a towering model you cannot be as thin either unless it's your natural shape which is highly unlikely because if it was you would be strutting down the catwalk scowling instead of reading this book. Discover *your* ideal shape, your optimum self, and in doing so uncover your bliss. You will be far less perturbed and far happier.

Much of our distress is caused by unreal expectations based on subterfuge and lies and the abuse of modern technology. Luscious star Kate Winslett has a perfect Libran body. Who can forget the sight of the curvaceous beauty soaring over the ocean wrapped in the arms of Leonardo di Caprio in the blockbuster Titanic? When Kate did a photo shoot for GQ magazine she was shocked to see that her body had been airbrushed to be more angular, long and lean than she actually was.

Who in their right mind would tamper with Kate and decide they could improve on it with some perverted ideal of beauty. Well done Kate for taking action which forced the magazine to issue an apology. What has our world come to when it plays God and tries to improve on his work? No wonder the rest of us are struggling. Weight is a complex issue with no easy answer and we are left with two fundamental truths.

1. DIETS DON'T WORK BECAUSE IF THEY DID WE WOULD ALL BE SLIM BY NOW.

Recent figures show that over 85% of women and 60% of men have dieted during their lifetime, with very little success. Interesting statistics because in Australia 60% of men are classified as overweight compared to 40% of women, which just goes to show that women are much conscious of their looks and men really don't give a hoot. On a recent episode of Oprah where she discussed her recent weight gain, her guest was a man who was the biggest loser of all time on the show The Biggest Loser. The unfortunate man had gained back over half his massive weight loss and looked as if he was returning to his original starting point. The man obviously enjoyed his food and like most of us, did not revel in exercise and restriction. Did he overeat? Probably. Was he happier when he was slim? Who knows? There's the dilemma ... enjoy and pay the price or deprive to live up to other's expectations.

2. WE WERE NOT ALL MEANT TO BE SLIM.

Until we accept this truth we will be miserable and in a state of constant emotional turmoil. We need to understand that the diet trade bolsters a thriving industry that is worth billions of dollars and feeds off our insecurity. There are some reputable organizations like Weight Watchers that boast good results because they are supportive and educate people to alter faulty eating habits and ultimately lead a better lifestyle. They help people to determine who they essentially are and become their very best and there can be no better goal than that.

Alas like the previous lady I am one of their early dropouts. I was not keen on the necessity to measure or think about food or stray from the foods that gave me pleasure. Food that I had grown up with and loved, those 'feel good' dishes of my youth. So if you join me among the ranks of the hopeless dieter please take heart. Love the real you. However if you have packed on the pounds to the point of discomfort or ill health then it's time to act and return to your central balanced core.

There are many reasons why we end up carrying excess weight and I offer what I believe to be the main causes. The list is by no means complete because weight is a complicated and challenging issue.

1. *Overeating.* Our world is full of rich and tempting food which tastes as good as it smells, feels and looks. It's delicious, so how are we mere mortals supposed to resist? The trend to upsize portions is counterproductive. Our stomachs expand along with our appetites and we become bigger, so as hard as it may be try to resist the temptation.

2. *The backlash effect.* Demanding that people stop eating while enticing them with wonderful food and then deriding them for doing so, when the rest of the population gets away with it, only causes extreme resentment and overeating. Large people are already excluded from many of society's delights and so to deny them of the last of those pleasures, food, is as distasteful and disheartening as it is unfair.

3. *Sluggish metabolism* caused by body type, health issues, family background, medication and genetics. Changes like puberty, childbirth, hysterectomy or menopause cause a metabolic shift that can have a huge impact on our weight. Age alters us. Exercise will not impact in a long lasting way for those who are not physically predisposed to it.

4. *Body type.* Some people are born big and beautiful and no amount of starvation or deprivation will alter their astrological or genetic makeup. This is a fact we should be grateful for. Each person is blessed with a unique imprint that ensures the diversity of our world, preventing the presence of a thin, controlling robotic master race.

5. *Inappropriate and unhealthy diet.* It is vital to identify the food that matches your body type and ancestral eating habits. Choose food that does not produce an allergic effect or cause bloating or other distress. Food that doesn't harm you but instead wishes you well.

The current ads produced for American TV in their anti obesity campaign are confronting and compelling, so much so that they may cause us to turn away and defeat their own purpose. However they are a shocking reminder of what we are actually ingesting in our body. That sugary, thirst quenching soda takes on a whole new unsavory dimension when we actually see what it is doing to our body. They come to us disguised, and so we need to be more aware and in control.

6. *Additives, pesticides and preservatives.* The very words imply that they are adding weight to our bodies, killing us off or at the very least embalming us. It's called getting fat without really trying. It's an impossible task to completely avoid them but increase your awareness, use your glasses while out shopping and do the best you can, that's if you can wade through the multitude of numbers that are so small on the packaging then have to be a Russian spy to decipher the code.

So if you don't want to end up like some poor chap who went to a Caribbean getaway on holiday and instead of coming back with a coconut carved souvenir, came back with a pair of full blown breasts he procured after eating some estrogen laden fried chicken, then I suggest you stick to natural products. If you can find any! For all you flat as a pancake girls, before you flock to the Caribbean to chomp on a bucket of steaming hot chicken, I suggest you stick to the implant option in case you get a dud hen and return home instead with two poached eggs!

Now let's take one last look at diet from a fatty perspective. Why has fat got such a bad reputation and why are we so frantic to get rid of it? The mere mention of the word is enough to make a grown woman shiver and a burly man with a saggy belly grab another beer to drown his sorrows. But is fat really so bad for you? Why has fat acquired such a bad wrap and why exactly does it exist, if only to plague society and terrify most of the population with its fleshy existence?

Personally I just don't get it. Sure, an overload of fat may look unsightly and wrinkle and wobble and squelch but there are worse things in life than a floppy arm or a floury muffin top. Would that we had more pressing issues to deal with than staring into a mirror and finding fault with ourselves. Plastic surgeons surely would agree that there is a big difference between a genuine problem that needs fixing and an inflicted dose of insecurity that convinces us we are unworthy.

Among other things, ill health is blamed on fat and indeed too much of a good thing, or a bad one, works against our wellbeing. But doesn't fat have its purposes? Surely there's a reason it exists. In reality fat performs important structural and metabolic functions and forms a category of lipids that are important for life. Edible animal fats are butter, lard, ghee and fish oil. Fish oil is consumed in capsule form by many people and has been found to have important healing properties, all those vital nourishing omegas.

Even plants have fats, many of which are good for us and essential for our health. Edible plant fats include peanut, sunflower, sesame, coconut, soya bean, olive and vegetable oils. Some fats are saturated while others are unsaturated. Some are better than others for us but fat is a fat by any other name. If in doubt, reach out for expert advice for guidance in this complex area.

Fat is vital to our wellbeing, a point that is not often raised. Vitamins A, D, E and K are fat soluble and can only be absorbed, digested and transported in conjunction with fats. Essential fatty acids are an important requirement in our diet. Fats provide us with energy, promote optimum cell function and help maintain healthy skin and hair. They also perform other important roles, like maintaining correct body temperature and insulating the body organs against shock.

Yes, fat has picked up a bad wrap over the years and supposedly is the major cause of a host of illnesses yet it also serves as a useful buffer against a host of diseases. When a toxic substance, chemical or biotic, reaches an unsafe level in the bloodstream, the body can dilute the offending substance by storing it in the fat tissue, so protecting the vital organs until the toxin can be excreted by the body safely.

To attempt to remove fat entirely from the body is unhealthy and there are purposes to it that no doubt have yet to be uncovered. Recent research has revealed that t-cells from belly fat can be harvested to heal heart problems. This procedure has been used on animals for some time. I watched the news fascinated as a stunning snow leopard from Sydney Zoo underwent surgery to remove t-cells from its tummy fat to inject into its damaged arthritic leg, a limb essential to its wellbeing. Yes, fat does have its purposes that go beyond extracting butt fat to plump up your cheeks or jowls. It might just surprise you in the end so don't think of fat as an unsightly lump or bump, but rather as an unlikely friend.

It is far better to be happy and at peace with yourself than to diet, be miserable and in a constant state of hunger, denial, frustration or obsession, all of which will deplete your life force much quicker than fat. The reality is that you may be exactly the way you were born to be, in which case all the slimming tea from China will have no effect. You were not put on this earth to suffer. Circumstances arise in life that cause us pain and we should not add to it unnecessarily. If the stress of trying to alter yourself to match some unrealistic ideal is greater than the stress placed on your body, mind or spirit by the effort or denial, then leave it alone. Instead delight in who you are because in truth you are delightful.

CONSCIOUS LIVING

Now that we have identified fat as a strange bedfellow, an ally of sorts, what should we make of it? Can we regard it differently, not see it as the enemy that has caused us unending years of anguish. Thinking back over all those strained times when I tried to banish it from my system brings an unhealthy flush to my cheeks and the sorry scent of defeat.

My last attempt at dieting was at the urging of a specialist, who 'recommended' that I lose weight for health reasons. I was determined to succeed for it was no longer about vanity but rather my health that was at stake. Why I was so optimistic after all my efforts over the past forty years had amounted to zilch remains unclear. Still I was fired with enthusiasm, determined that this time would be different.

For months I ate a small bowl of oatmeal for breakfast, salad lunches and low calorie fish dinners with little appeal. I was almost self righteous as I ordered salad instead of my regular sandwich. I suffered the entire time, feeling queasy and ill, because the diet didn't agree with me. I became an emotional time bomb. It just wasn't fair and I felt cheated as I watched a battalion of thin people in the mall gorge food as if they were competing in a burger eating marathon or sitting down for the Last Supper. These were no saints but rather ordinary people who ate what they wanted without an obvious care or worry in the world.

After the frustration and anger came the resentment. Why could others eat what they liked while I had to watch every morsel I put in my mouth? I hated the fact that once again my life revolved around food, or more precisely the lack of it. Diets had taken up far too many of my years and I didn't want to waste another thought on food. I just wanted to enjoy life and to be happy.

Then when I went to Hawaii on vacation I watched in disbelief as plane loads of Japanese ate their way through Hungry Jacks like a horde of deranged locusts and then polished off a truckload of Baskin and Robbins Ice Cream in one sitting. Their appetite was voracious. It didn't make sense. This entire nation of people were reed thin, ate like truckers and got up to no more exercise than clicking a camera shutter or making a beeline for the Revlon counter at Long's Drug Store. I burned up far more calories trying to get out of their way. Apart from being demoralized, their actions reinforced my belief that many people get away with overeating and no exercise without getting fat.

Several months later I returned to the specialist's office for my weigh in. I dreaded it because I sensed I had lost no weight. I was right, not an ounce. Months of going without food amounted to nothing. My doctor looked at me with disdain, convinced I was a closet eater. I looked at my specialist with disdain for wishing this upon me. He had no idea how much I had suffered and saw only numbers and not a soul in distress. To him I was not only overweight, I was weak willed and incompetent, a failure at best. I wanted to remind him of his HIPPO-CRATIC OATH. To love, honor and obey his patients regardless of their weight, faulty DNA or fatty tendencies. I fought off the urge to ask for a referral to a plastic surgeon for HIPPO-SUCTION. I knew that no amount of sucking or slurping would relieve me of my fat. It was mine to keep, to love, honor and obey. I was stuck with it and it with me.

I sought comfort in my doctor's office. I was a blubbering mess as I lay my head down on his desk. My doctor is a gem. He has been my support for the last thirty years and without him I would not have lasted through my ordeals. He reminds me of a kind cuddly koala. 'I tried,' I wailed, 'but I haven't lost an ounce.' I didn't relate how humiliating it was getting on the scales at the specialist's office and his incriminating look. I resented feeling like a failure once again.

'It's not easy,' my doctor replied, because he too had tried losing weight without success. Food was a comfort for us both. As a writer who stared at the computer screen all day I longed for inspiration. It came when I wandered into the kitchen and opened the fridge. My doctor was a man of compassion who faced heartbreak each day. There were difficult diagnoses and sad passages and he knew how transient life could be. At the end of the day he just wanted to go home to the pleasure of a good meal, a loving spouse and a warm bed.

'Why did I bother,' I sniffed, wanting to grab a nearby syringe and siphon off the excess pounds, wrap the blood pressure monitor around my neck and squeeze or self mutilate with his thermometer.

'You didn't lose weight but you didn't *gain* any either,' he said, with the wisdom of a prophet. 'You maintained your *correct* weight.'

If the way you are now is the way you were meant to be then you must learn to accept it and love who you are, despite the mountain of pressure to change. You must never, ever allow your spirit to be broken because without it your body is useless and cannot function. You are not accountable to anyone. Not your partner, your parents, your friends, the magazine editors or the invisible masses that make up society. The only person you have to please is yourself, so ease the pressure. You are carrying tons of weight accumulated from other people's comments and society's unreal expectations. Shed it and get on with your life.

You don't have to feel heavy any more. Become more conscious of the way you live. Rather than diet make healthy, sound choices so that you can be the optimum you. Bring pleasure into your life so that the joy you experience is not all centered on the eating but also on the telling, the feeling, the expression and the sharing. You have so much to give but you cannot do so until you give back to yourself.

Now to lighten the load and help you understand the way of the cosmos, I present a guide to potential astrological trouble spots. So if you were to pack on the pounds this is where they would land. There is order in divine chaos, so we start at the top with the first sign Aries then work our way down. Each sign correlates to a different part of the body.

Aries rules the head, so it's tempting to say that Arians have a big head, an even bigger ego and are rather selfish. The head is their most vulnerable area and they are subject to stress related migraines. One of my former beaus was a tall Aries with a Pisces Moon, with his head always in the clouds. He was continually hitting his head, scraping it on overhanging signs and bumping into doorways. Fortunately for him he was in another head space so he barely noticed.

Taurus governs the throat so watch out for any nasty goiter or a sluggish thyroid which can pile on the weight and make you top-heavy. The effect of Taurus extends to the chest which is usually large and impressive, and the feisty bull makes for big busted women or men with a stubborn streak. You may attempt to reduce them, like my friend Beverly, but alas they often just grow back like ripe melons in May.

Gemini rules the chest and particularly the lungs which is their vulnerable area. Geminis rarely pack on the pounds because they're too busy dashing about and puffing away on cigarettes which can lead to their untimely demise. The more disciplined ones can have breathing difficulties like asthma and pollen allergies through no fault of their own. Remain calm, resist the urge to run off and take a deep breath.

Cancerians are rather short and a little fleshy. Their sign rules the stomach and other digestive organs, like the liver, pancreas and gall bladder. Little crabs can be round like their namesake and pack on the pounds round their middle. Men are prone to beer bellies and women to broadening waistlines. Problems arise from poor digestion, often the result of emotional issues that impact poorly on their eating habits.

Leos are larger than life. Everything's big about them. Their voice, their personalities but most noticeably their hair which they love to fluff up. If there's such a thing as fat hair they've got it. They also have ample regal chests like a strutting lion and can purr on command. Leo rules the heart and they are big hearted people. Avoid too much swaggering and blustering about because it may just take its toll and others may get really annoyed in your shadow.

My crazy Leo friend Roxy has a grand bosom which she loves to show off and masses of wavy auburn hair. While she was touring the Orangutan Reserve in Borneo with a travel group a giant ape took a liking to her, convinced he'd found his ideal mate. He began whooping away in the trees and beating his chest in rapture, before swooping down to capture her. She barely made it through the gate with the ranger to escape his amorous clutches! She never went near the jungle again.

Virgo is the virgin of the zodiac but she is endowed with fecund hips and a rounded bottom so she won't stay that way for very long. Despite that fabulous booty, Virgo rules the intestines and bowels so don't put too pressure on them because you may live to regret it. If the flatulence doesn't get you then the burst appendix definitely will.

Libra as the goddess Venus reborn has the classic hourglass figure and if she packs on the pounds she is fortunate because it will distribute evenly into a mass of heavenly curves. Plump, with long shining hair, fluttering eyelashes and a heart shaped face she will be hard to resist. You can never have too much of a good thing but alas her kidneys may suffer because of her excesses, so tone it down a bit.

Scorpios are the Gothics of the zodiac and would love to paint the world black. The sign rules the reproductive organs but I'm not sure how you would judge if you had obese ovaries or tubby tubes. Scorpios burn off weight with their unusual tantric sexual practices and by repeating OM till it hurts. They may also discard some extra baggage by putting some deathly curse on you, so stay well out of their way.

Sagittarians have an athlete's stance and strong sturdy thighs. They may be mistaken for a horse from behind because of their strong equine flanks so check out the front before you attempt to ride them. When they stack on the weight their upper legs look like two Weiner sausages stuffed into tights but they go great with mustard and relish.

Lean Capricorn rules the knees which are weak and rather knobby. Their problem areas include their teeth, skin and bones. With their poor circulation they feel the cold and their weight comes from all the blankets, sweaters, gloves and beanies they pile on top of themselves to keep warm. Anything to avoid paying the gas or electricity bill or to admit to being vaguely vulnerable.

With Aquarius weight comes from their ponderous minds. They think far too much for their own good. This makes them top heavy which is not ideal because their weak point is their spindly ankles. Take care when you walk with them because their ankles give way at the most awkward moments and you have to keep picking them up off the pavement. At least they're light so you don't do yourself an injury.

Pisces are bloated. They have problems with fluid retention so their overflowing lymphatic system needs a good drainage. Massage could squelch it out of them but unfortunately with the first glass of water it will flood through their bodies and just rearrange. They'd prefer it was gin. The sign rules the feet so apart from fatty corns and bunions, they would prefer to have flippers rather than feet and waddle through life or go for a swim in the ocean and never come back.

Now that you understand where your problem areas are, consider the following tips to maintain your ideal weight. Not for losing weight because the very term implies failure. You're no loser, you're a WINNER. There is no place for negatives in your vocabulary and no room for defeat. This is a win, win situation. As you discover the real you, you will become more beautiful, confident, and more comfortable in your own skin. You will be successful because you believe you can be and that you deserve it. Others will respond to the change in you, feeding the fabulous flames of fire within. Whatever form they take.

TOP TIPS
FOR STAYING TIP TOP

You should always strive to be your personal best. If you believe you overeat or are carrying too much weight to feel healthy or comfortable, a subject strictly between your libido and your Higher Self, then do something about it. Your aim is to improve, not deprive, yourself. Remain positive and be optimistic. The following are some tips that might just help you along the way and lead you in the right direction.

First you need some *inspiration*, something to kick start you into action and make a difference. Change is a tricky business and as the old saying goes, 'you can't teach an old dog new tricks.' That's particularly the case with a tubby old hound that loves chewing on his mangled well-loved bone. Don't bury his bone where he can't find it but rather give him some new toys to play with and divert his attention elsewhere.

Let's try the old fridge trick, with a twist. Take a picture of Paris Hilton or Bobby Dazzler, or any other idol you don't aspire to be, and draw a moustache and horns on them and stick it on your fridge with a monkey magnet. Now find a photo of you at your best. Not your most unrealistic or thin, but your personal *best*. The one with a big smile on your face, at a time when you were content and truly happy.

Stick that on your fridge for true inspiration. Choose an animal to stand by you, one you identify with or that makes you laugh or inspires you. Place its photo on the fridge next to you. That photo will be a constant reminder that we are all created differently, with our own character and tastes. When we choose extreme diets or ones unsuited to us, they damage us. You would never give a zebra a raw steak or a bunch of grass to a tiger. If we eat what does not suit us then we suffer.

Atkin's protein diet was detrimental for many because people need carbohydrates, an essential food group as part of a well balanced diet. Our optimum diet may be shaped by the tribe from which we are descended. Their staple diet over the centuries determines what foods suit our digestive system. My tribe was into cake and candy. You probably already know from experience what is good for you and the foods or allergens that stress your system.

Over the years I had a number of allergy tests to assess why I had problems with my digestion. Blood tests, needle pricks, hair analysis and even computerized acupuncture assessments. Allergies are hard to determine because they manifest in two ways. The most obvious is an immediate severe reaction when we ingest them. Alcohol makes my mouth burn and I cannot swallow it. The smell of coffee sends me into a tailspin and hot foods like ginger, onion, capsicum and chili make my taste buds explode and then blast their way through my intestines. Like many others, I learned the hard way what foods to avoid at all costs.

One friend ended up in a hospital emergency room after a night out a Chinese restaurant with a dose of MSG. Her airways closed up and she nearly died. Peanuts send some folk into immediate shock and in one extreme case some unfortunate lass died after kissing her boyfriend who had eaten a peanut butter sandwich several hours earlier. Dairy allergies often cause 'glue ear' which I discovered while assessing children referred to me for learning or behavioral difficulties. A runny nose was an immediate giveaway and even though the problem manifested as an emotional one, its base was purely physical. What child can concentrate or sit still when they can't hear? As a result they suffer from a short attention span because the rest of the world is a blur to them.

Such allergic reactions result from the food we crave. Foods that we love but don't love us back. Many children with glue ear or associated problems admit to drinking many glasses of milk each day. Although dairy products are seen as healthy they can unfortunately do more harm than good for some, especially when consumed in excess. Chocolate might be your passion but it could give you a headache or tax your liver. Some people are gluten intolerant but without bread they feel uneasy. They crave it even though it may bloat their stomach or stack on the weight. An addiction, whatever its form, cause or effect, is a hard habit to kick.

We often drink without conscious thought. It is one of the easiest things to improve in our diet because generally drink does not provide as much comfort as food, unless you're an alcoholic or coffee addict. Fizzy drinks are relatively easy to cut out or reduce and after a while you won't miss them. My preferred drink is lemonade but now I ask for iced water with a slice of lemon and it's just as good. Diet sodas are stacked with chemicals and many 'health' drinks are brimming with sugar and calories, so choose the low fat kind. Best of all are bottled water and fresh vegetable and fruit juice. Despite their best intentions most people don't include enough vegetables in their diet. The easiest and most nourishing way to do so is in fresh juice. Try carrot, apple and celery juice for a refreshing, healthy break or whatever suits your taste.

Avoid mindless eating. Going to the movies can be a 3D experience and we saturate all of our senses to fully immerse ourselves. We stare up at the big screen rapt, our mouths chomping on handfuls of popcorn. Which we wash down with a large Pepsi and sweeten with a huge candy bar or a jumbo box of sweet treats. The cinemas cash in big time, the portions are massive and then they ask if you would like to upgrade for a mere $2 more.

NO, NO, NO. Never go for the super size upgrades unless you're hanging out in the cinema with a gang or you too will become super sized. As a measure of discipline, imagine the popcorn popping into little balls of cellulite on your ample thighs right in front of Brad Pitt or George Clooney as they stare down at you from the silver screen. That is not to say you shouldn't enjoy the experience but in moderation.

Then there's everyone's best friend, TV. How many nights have you eaten in front of it, as if it's your family which unfortunately it often substitutes to be? No, you're not having dinner with the gals at Wisteria Lane, who wouldn't know a grilled chop if they tripped over it, or sharing lunch with Dr. Phil as he mulls over your issues. Instead you're eating without thinking which means you won't be satisfied and will want more. Be content but not mindless. To prevent grazing at night avoid those programs that will have you running for food. The Hallmark channel could be a problem if you're sentimental and need to eat while you cry. We're talking tubs of vanilla ice cream here, drooling with lots of thick caramel syrup and chopped nuts on top.

Music is great. Put on something that will prompt you to dance to ensure that you get your daily exercise. Whatever does it for you - belly dancing, ballroom, swing or rapping with the broom. I personally like to tango but my unfortunate cat is not a willing partner. Dance, and then put on some happy music to uplift your spirits. Dean Martin does it for me. He sounds like he's sozzled on Chianti and is in a permanent state of bliss. Who can fail to share his joy when he sings Volare, and tells you how his happy heart sings? If it's just before bedtime and you don't want to snack avoid the tracks, 'When the Moon hits your eye like a big pizza pie' and 'Hey brothers, pour the wine.' Then put on New Age, 'Dribbling Waterfalls of the Amazon' and drift off to sleep.

Danger foods. We all have them. Foods that once you start eating, you cannot stop until the whole lot's demolished. These are your culinary Achilles heel. Avoid them at all costs. Mine are creamy lemon filled tarts, in a packet of six. They're meant to last three days but they don't last three hours. They melt in the mouth, slide down the pleasure chute of your throat straight into your willing stomach. One of my friends confesses to eating a whole jar of chocolate covered peanuts in one sitting, another devours a full container of praline ice cream. Those with a savory taste crave deep fried chicken or a huge packet of potato chips. Go past these danger foods in the supermarket with steely resolve and gritted teeth. Better still bypass that aisle entirely or else you will be forced to live with the consequences.

Here's a handy hint in reverse psychology. Go on to the next best thing. Something you quite like but do not crave and then buy a cart full. Go ahead and fill up an entire shelf in your cupboard with your treats. Sound's weird but it works. By doing so, you transform its status from a forbidden pleasure and the glut will put you off. We only crave what we can't have. This strategy also protects you from the 'empty cupboard syndrome'. It's a strange phenomenon that happens when we clear out all the treats from our pantry and suddenly feel deprived.

In the middle of the night when your body is reeling from a sugar shortage, you freak out. You go the cupboard desperate for anything to satisfy your craving. Alas nothing. You give up and go back to what you were doing. Ten minutes later, you get up again to examine the cupboard. Surely you've missed something. A stale packet of crackers, or even a few crumbs. You repeat the pattern until you're crawling up the wall, with your nails leaving groove marks on the cupboard door.

NEVER put yourself in that situation because you'll resort to desperate measures, rifling through all the frayed take away menus in your kitchen drawer desperate for anything that's open at midnight. To prevent late night jitters, fill your stomach with protein. After a grilled fish or omelet you will not be hungry for a long time. Listen to your body. Empty carbohydrates and sugars are just that. Empty, and they won't satisfy you. You will come back for more.

Let fresh fruit satisfy your desire for sweets in a nutritious way and if you must keep nibbling have a packet of sugar free candy in the desk draw, or in your purse or pocket. The new fruit ones taste good although I'm not sure what has gone into them to make them so tangy. Keep a packet of cookies in the cupboard just in case, to stop you ending up in blood sugar or emotional distress late at night. Some people prefer a few almonds, or an assortment of nuts and seeds, which while highly nutritious are also high in calories. They also present a problem for the dentally challenged who could do themselves an injury while munching.

Smell excites the palate, like the lingering aroma of freshly baked bread, roasting coffee beans or hot donuts. Instead of giving in to the temptation, I buy a bunch of fresh roses and inhale their delicate scent as I shop through the mall. It's a pleasant distraction. A good hint is to brush your teeth immediately after eating. The taste of food excites our taste buds and so we swing from sweet to sour, and back again. Once the taste has been wiped off your tongue, and erased from your palate, you lose the desire to eat. Spray your home with essential oils, geranium, rose or lavender, so any lingering food scent is replaced by a calm soothing perfume. Fill your life with pleasure of different kinds.

We come home late at night tired and wiped out from the stresses of modern life. Frazzled from the ride on the train or bus, the hoards of people and traffic, and the strains of work we are worn out and often alone. Food becomes our best friend, our ray of light in what is perceived by some as a harsh, dark world. It also comforts those of us who are overrun with kids, noise and too much stimulation. We wander off to our inner sanctum where we can be alone. Eating is a Zen act where we are in control. It is a rare quiet moment and equally fulfilling.

To uncover your bliss, explore other options. Find out what makes you happy, complete and content. My house is filled with scented flowers, music floats through each room, my cat puts a smile on my face, my writing ignites my imagination, my friends support me, the sea captivates me, the stars inspire me with their beauty and their wisdom. My faith carries me through the long nights and helps me turn the darkness into the light. Sharing it with you makes it all worthwhile.

WHAT'S THIS
ABOUT EXERCISE?

'I'm in shape. Round is a shape isn't it?' Anon.

There are those gung ho sorts who like nothing better than climbing the Himalayas followed by a fleet of Sherpas or jumping out of a plane attached to nothing but some spindly cords and a large hanky. There are also types who like to go up in a hot air balloon or drive motorbikes at phenomenal speeds across impossible distances. That's not me.

I'm one of those sedate people who like nothing more than to sit in muted sunlight by an open fireside with a mug of hot chocolate and read a good book. To meet friends and have a leisurely chat over a pot of tea and a slice of cake, or indulge in a pleasant walk in the park followed by a relaxing massage. That's more like it, much more refined.

Expecting everyone to exercise each day on a treadmill is as unrealistic as it is unrewarding. Animals like to preserve their energy. Lions hang around under a bush in the shade waiting for an unsuspecting antelope to wander by and let the ladies of the pride do all the hard work, rising only for a good feed and a relaxing stroll after dinner. Most tree dwellers are content to hang off a dangly branch, scrambling down to earth only to escape the occasional scorpion or snake or to harass a passing echidna with a stick dipped in an ant dune.

Similarly to animals most people find contrived exercise both boring and a waste of time. They would prefer to be doing something far more valuable like looking after their family, discovering a cure for cancer, writing their autobiography, trading on Wall Street or simply having fun. There are lots of distractions and purposes in the world.

In addition many people have limitations that make it painful and even impossible to exert themselves or to even get up off the couch. Ask someone who suffers from arthritis or fibromyalgia to zumba themselves stupid, or a person with chronic fatigue to attend an aerobic class. Yes, I'm sure you'll argue that they could do a gentler class of tai chi, yoga or Pilates. With some people that's true and it helps them but in others it's very stressful and only aggravates their condition.

As a result of my surgery it's painful for me to raise my arms so even moderate forms of exercise are difficult. I forced myself to swim to loosen my muscles but it worsened my condition so in the end I just let it be, trying not to feel like a failure or endure any further pain. Walking is my salvation and long strolls, preferably in nature, give me great pleasure. I adore dancing and music still has the power to stir me but after a minute or so of twirling, I'm worn out and sore. It's my greatest regret that those days of my wild youth are over but at least I can still dance in my mind and my spirit can still boogie and jive.

There's an art to finding your center of gravity and discovering what your body is capable of and loves to the point of madness. We each march to a different drummer and to a different tune. There are patterns in the universe and each sign has its own preference. When it comes to exercise here are some winning tips to get your sign moving. Remember we are each our own unique mix of planets and signs so modify the forms of movement until you find your own groove.

ARIES likes to get down and dirty. They love to tackle, scrimmage, whack, thump and are the risk takers of the zodiac. Football, grid iron, jet skis, rally cross, roller blading, skate boarding, skiing or car racing, this planet of action likes things fast and even more furious.

TAURUS is much too refined to get in the mud or to squander precious energy. As Taurus rules the throat, its people like to sing. They belong in a choir or performing on the stage or in a soul band. They also like to shop for expensive and tasteful objects, so for

146

exercise I recommend they warble and sing while flitting around the gift shops of the mall.

GEMINIS, the twins, do best when they're twisting their body into two to best resemble their other half. Pilates could be just the go, or yoga, so they can stand on their head and see what the other half looks like. Their alter ego likes nothing better than to spend its day in the library, so they can exercise by balancing a pile of books on their head while assuming a yoga pose in the out of print section.

CANCER is a reclusive sign that withdraws into its shell when threatened. It's hard to motivate because it's hypersensitive and prefers to mope in the dark on a secluded beach. Preferably motionless. It's a water sign so if it can be induced to actually enter the water, it could attempt some delicate synchronized swimming with the rest of its crustacean friends. Most days it chooses to burrow all alone in the sand.

LEO loves to shine. A fire sign, Leo burns energy by getting its hair streaked or getting its claws buffed up and polished bright crimson. It likes to embellish them with flashy florals, sparkling diamonds or wild geometrics to assert its clawing rights. A Leo needs to be center stage so it can roar loudly and flounce about in some theatrical drama.

VIRGOS are hypochondriacs. They are seen roaming hospital corridors in an apparent daze or downing bottles of pills or vitamins. They are a whiz in the office so they could burn off fat if they were let loose in a twenty storey building and asked to reorganize the space. They are also great at vacuuming, a wonderful fat burner, and are closet hoarders. Just ask them to get rid of stuff and watch them meltdown.

LIBRAS are averse to anything that makes them sweat. Doused in sweet perfume, they don't mind taking a stroll as long as the view is scenic or they will reach somewhere worth getting to. I love to amble through the park near my home smelling the delicate blooms but if you really want to see me work up a sweat then watch me sprint the mile to the nearest KFC. Massage is their exercise of choice because they get to feel good while someone else is working up a sweat!

SCORPIOS are into all things exotic. In the body it rules the sexual organs and on a world map, India. A Scorpionic delight, the country abounds in temples that worship the *yoni* and the *lingam*, the female and male private parts. Scorpios choose the best way to burn off calories … tantric sex. After several hours of hot love they may also belly dance around their partner or handcuff them firmly to the bed.

SAGITTARIANS are the leapers and bounders of the zodiac. They love to use their long legs for the triple jump, to hurdle across a field or to vault over high bars. Nothing thrills them more than a jog or to bounce around a tennis or squash court. As they're also into travel, they would be excited to run a marathon across the Gobi desert or compete in a wild horse race against the tribesmen of the Kalahari.

CAPRICORNS love to scale things, preferably mountains. With their sturdy hoofs, they like nothing better than to clamber over rocks and go for long bush walks where they can nibble on some berries and rest on the grass. Hopefully they will not lose their way and require a whole squad of emergency workers or a rescue helicopter to come find them when they've fallen down a rocky ledge in the noonday sun.

AQUARIUS. Well, you'd be lucky to get one to go out in the sun at all, they're averse to it. They suffer from weak ankles and that's their excuse anyway. They also guard their pale complexion, a legacy from hours of mental exercise spent indoors reading books, playing chess or computer games, and any other technological diversions.

I suspect the South Korean guy who died after playing online computer games for fifty hours with scarcely a break was an Aquarian. He passed away at twenty eight, on his first Saturn return, but by this age the guy should have known better. As for the unfortunate Ms Strange from California who also died at twenty eight after drinking copious liters of water in a ridiculous radio competition, there's a possibility she was a Pisces. They're heavily into water but prefer a beverage laced with something stronger.

PISCES are lovers of the sea and like nothing better than to wile away hours in the tub or in the ocean. They can be puffy and wrinkly but make good marathon swimmers, and also excellent barmen who love to juggle empty bottles over their head. As Neptune rules music, Pisces like to dance preferably in some romantic setting overlooking the ocean at Diamond Head to the sound of Hawaiian guitars.

It's all very well to stay fit but for some folk that means keeping the mind challenged rather than the body. It would be ludicrous to have suggested that brilliant Einstein run around the block or dare waste a moment of his precious time. The great composers Lennon and McCartney were air signs, Libra and Gemini, and I can't see either of them jogging or bouncing for hours on a trampoline because their creative juices were channeled into the thing they loved most, music. Bob Dylan, Elton John, or Andrew Lloyd Weber don't look to be the type to swim the English Channel, just as Cassius Clay couldn't easily write a sonnet. Different strokes for different folks, thankfully.

People who are *too* much into their head can neglect their body. We must remain conscious that our bodies need to be looked after and replenished with good food, fresh air, movement and sunshine. Man cannot live by thought alone, rather he needs to take time to go smell the roses. The reverse is also true. Too much exercise can put you at increased risk. While heavy people sometimes require knee or hip replacements at an elderly age, young active ones need them much sooner. By putting too much strain on their knees, ligaments and joints, they wear them out. Active sports can cause a multitude of injuries, from broken bones to more serious, permanent damage to the spine.

While there is a non stop onslaught about the cost accrued to the medical system caused by the 'obesity epidemic' we seem to discount costs resulting from careless accidents triggered by speed, risk, sport and foolish decisions. These costs are rarely mentioned as if they are somehow justified in the name of healthier pursuits or are in some way not self inflicted. The opposite is true yet it is not viewed from the same perspective nor is the element of blame as blatant or pronounced.

It is also claimed that obese people are more at risk than thin ones of dying from health related issues like diabetes, heart attack and other such complications. A report in the Journal of the American Medical Association shows otherwise. After a twenty year study on adults over sixty years of age it was found that the more fit a person is, regardless of waist size or level of obesity, the longer they can expect to live. In fact, obese people who were fit had a lower risk of all-cause mortality, than unfit normal or lean people. It appears that fit rather than fat is the crucial factor in life expectancy. Shooting down the myth that overweight people will self-destruct and bring the planet down right along with them. Here's another myth shot down in flames. A recent study shows that eating chocolate at least five times a week REDUCES the risk of heart attack. Not only because dark chocolate is rich in antioxidants but also I guess because it makes you feel good.

There are no guarantees in life and things don't always work out as planned. A young man in my local health food store was a picture of glowing health. He ate only fresh food, regularly took vitamins and exercised a lot. One day after he had gone for surf, he was carrying his surfboard to his car when his heart gave way and he dropped dead. Who can understand the intricacies of divine wisdom or respond to impossible questions that have no answers? To define what is 'fit' is complicated because it is as much a state of mind as of the body. To be healthy implies that all layers of a person are in harmony – the body, mind, spirit and soul. That is true health, health at its best.

A life worth living must be an enjoyable one, full of promise and personal growth. If your life is lacking or unfulfilled, or you feel depressed or hopeless, turn it around. Fitness is within reach if you keep your goals realistic. It can be achieved by only thirty minutes of exercise, five days a week. So walk to the station, cavort around the telegraph poles, meander through the park, sprint around the supermarket with your trolley, dance the salsa at your local club, chase your dog around the lake or pursue that 'hottie' around the water cooler at work but make sure it's consensual because your workmate or dog may take offence. Whatever does it for you, do it. And do it regularly.

THE MEEK SHALL INHERIT
THE EARTH

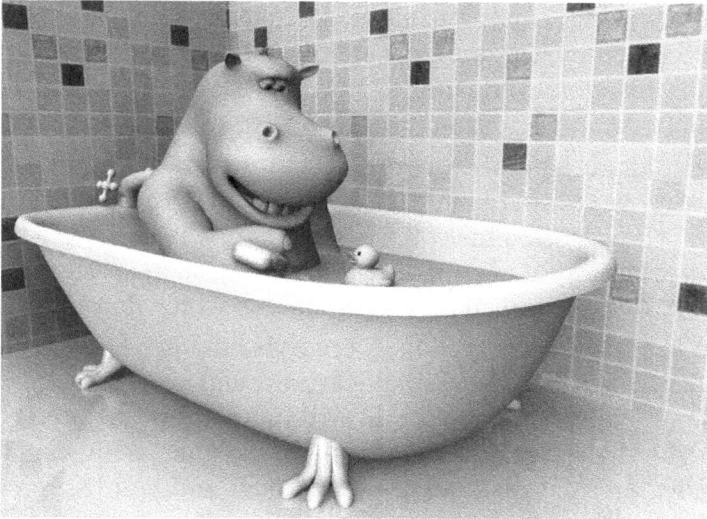

Here's the problem. The weighty planets are the 'nice' amenable planets and those born under their influence are generally a pleasant lot. They accept the status quo because they don't want to make waves, are not confident enough to confront it or to instigate change, or because they don't want to offend or hurt anyone other than themselves.

This allows the stroppy planets to take over. Here's how it works. Let's start with Mercury, a deceptive little planet. Positioned close to the Sun it's a cosmic flare waiting to happen. Blinded by the glare, we don't see it coming. Mercury is a difficult element to contain. Just drop it on the floor and watch it scatter all over. Then try putting it back together. Wanting to spread its influence, Mercury is not content to rule over one sign. It claims two signs, Gemini and Virgo.

151

Mercury is the planet of communication so Geminis love to gab. Placed in Virgo, Mercury is all about research preferably of the medical variety because the fastidious god is not keen on germs. Mercury is the slippery messenger god with wings on his feet so who knows what bugs he's picked up along the way. He can direct pigeons carrying important messages on the right path and bring down telephone wires and jam up switchboards in record time. He also rules the internet and the media which are the most crucial means of communication across the world.

Mercury is a bit of a trickster. He may distort things just to play games with your mind which the media have been accused of doing many times over. Gemini is the sign of the twins, so Mercury tends to suffer from a split personality. Plagued by such an identity crisis, the media sends us mixed messages most of which don't make sense.

When it comes to weight, Mercury's having a field day. It's got the bull by the horns, ploddy old Taurus, and won't let go. Beware because one day the enraged bull will jump out of the arena and rip him to shreds. Pick up a handful of weekly magazines and check out the features splashed all over the cover and you'll soon see the dilemma.

'Celebs true weight EXPOSED!' the headlines scream, along with some candid shots of dimpled buttocks, rolls of fat and double chins to sweeten the mix. Then there's 'Steal Posh's new diet' with diabolical ways to lose twenty pounds fast. On the cover of another issue is 'Refusing to Eat. Why these stars look so scary skinny.' The media is obsessed with body shape, as if no other issue exists in the world, and in doing so ensures that we become obsessed with it too.

Make up your mind! Too fat or too thin? Too robust or too skeletal? Ridiculous by-lines that can't possibly make sense even to the feeble or narrow minded. Like how some celebrity lost half her body weight. Read the small print and it appears she lost forty pounds which doesn't quite add up because the hefty lass certainly wasn't eighty pounds to begin with. Misleading, very misleading, and downright sneaky.

Imagine what the person behind this invisible hand who writes this stuff looks like. Is he some scrawny male with poxy skin who has nothing better to do than sit behind his office desk and bite his nails while thinking up horrid headlines? Has he got a giant chip on his shoulder and wants to share his misery or is he just trying to please his boss? One thing's for sure, he ain't no Adonis or potential boy genius because if he was he'd be elsewhere getting a life.

Then picture the gaunt editor nibbling on tossed basil leaves and a glass of soda with a slice of lemon as she pours over photos of cerebrally challenged women who would starve themselves all for the sake of a picture. The truth is most editors are just normal men or women who should know better, in terms of the damage they inflict.

'Have they gone too far or are they in total denial?' the blurb continues, with the words pasted over starlets who look as if they're on the brink of starvation. They obviously have gone too far but so have the magazines. What sort of crazed messages are they sending? It's a fine line between good health and dieting yourself into an early grave.

That's when Saturn steps in. This austere god is the master of wasting away and death, be it physical or symbolic. Mercury leads us to him, for according to mythology Mercury is the solemn guide of the dead, the Divine Herald who leads the souls down to their final home where the god Saturn is patiently waiting to scoop them into his hold.

With Saturn we must come to grips with the harsh realities of life. Saturn's into suffering and he likes to put us through the mill to toughen us up. Through the obstacles he presents and gritty hard work, we develop the qualities of self-discipline and determination. But he's one rigid and cold god so the lessons he hands us are difficult ones.

Capricorn is the sign that Saturn rules and it's not the most sympathetic of signs. Business minded, it's obsessed with money and status. People born under the sign can be tough on themselves and have no time for weaknesses in others. They don't suffer fools or laid back folk gladly and can't understand why you have weight issues when they're so in control. They could live on a sprig of parsley or meager rations, so why can't you? Capricorn friends meet you for lunch and arrive with two wrapped Wheat crackers scraped with flakes of tuna. Capricorns are old goats at heart, renowned for their strange eating habits. They can even digest a load of tin cans and get away with it.

Now add to the mix Aries, the god of War. Aries was a testy lad who was the son of the Greek gods Zeus and Hera, both of whom apparently detested him. It's a bit rough when both your parents can't stand you so I guess he was carrying a grudge which he decided to inflict on the whole world. Described as 'bloodstained, murderous and the curse of mortals,' Aries was a ruthless, vengeful god. On the battlefield he was accompanied by his sister Discord and her son Strife. Also lending their support were Terror, Trembling and Panic. Not a great bunch, but you'd certainly want them on your side in a face off.

The Romans, a military race of people, made Aries more heroic when they converted him into Mars, an invincible warrior who stood tall and proud in his shining armor. With such a formidable ruler, Aries folk like to whip you into shape and make the best personal trainers because most were Roman gladiators in a past lifetime. They probably scaled the Seven Hills of Rome while devouring a whole side of beef.

The next ruthless god to enter the fray is Uranus, the god of the sky. He came down at night to cover the earth and mate with the lovely Gaia. Unfortunately he hated the children she bore him, the dreaded titans, and imprisoned some deep within the earth. Gaia was not the type to lie down and take it so in revenge she carved a sickle out of rock and demanded her sons castrate him. Cronus, being the more malicious type, agreed and cut off his father's testicles.

Uranus was incensed and after prophesying that Cronus's sons would one day rise up to overthrow him he vowed to exact a terrible revenge. To prevent such a heinous fate, Cronus ate each of his sons. This was one dysfunctional family and did not make for healthy eating habits right from the start. An erratic god, Uranus rules over lightning, revolutions and all things sudden. His charges, the Aquarians of the world, are equally weird and eccentric but often in an endearing way. As for Cronus he moved to Rome and changed his name to Saturn.

Here's an alarming fact. The bossy planets, and the overpowering gods that rule them, have dominated our lives for too long. They have called the shots simply because they can and it's time for a sweeping change. The sweeter more docile signs must rise up in protest and refuse to accept the oppression or to be put down any longer.

Trouble is, the softer signs are happiest in their own private world and don't like or seek confrontation. Under pressure, water signs retreat. Cancerians crawl back into their shells by the light of the moon and become hypersensitive and hurt if slighted. Scorpios scowl and brood a lot before putting a Plutonic curse on the next mean person they come across. Pisceans are too gentle for revenge and instead turn their frustration onto themselves. They will drink, shoot up, wallow in music or watch Days of Our Lives until they self destruct and implode.

Charming Venus, personified in the beauteous signs of Taurus and Libra, does not want to say a bad word or offend and the lovely goddess is far too genteel to be brutally honest. She prefers to paint the world in colors of the rainbow and move into a mountain retreat surrounded by flowers and cooing doves, languishing about in flowing caftans, soft angora shawls and comfortable jersey knits, with all her fluffy pussycats. Far away from the lowly affairs of man.

Now, here's the thing. The gentle signs don't realize their own strength. Ruled by the big planets, they have infinite power waiting to be unleashed. With one stroke of his trident Neptune can cause the sea to rise up and engulf you, Pluto can drop a bomb, Jupiter will make you bankrupt, the moon will let you bleed to death, and worst of all Venus will make sure you don't get any action in the bedroom for a very, very long time. Not to mention the subterranean itch and genital warts.

So take heart and be brave. It's time for action. Stand up and be counted. Demand change. Insist that stores cater for *everyone* in equal measure and that clothes in larger sizes are glamorous and stylish, that images appear in magazines and the media that reflect an array of real people with all their individual quirks and qualities, that film and television portray all types of people in a positive and self affirming light. Demand that naturally larger people are recognized to be just as beautiful, just as worthy and just as desirable as anyone else.

Repeat it over and over again until you truly acknowledge and believe it. *Size is one of the last and nastiest forms of discrimination that exists in our society today.* It's rationalized in the guise of health but who exactly has the right to determine acceptable guidelines other than ourselves. We are governed by a sublime intelligence and without all the pressure to change and alter our looks, we can tap into its force.

By asserting your right to be the best that you were created to be, to revel in the inherent beauty bestowed upon you by a supreme benevolent force, you can influence the world to become a more tolerant, kinder, supportive, compassionate and accepting place. Strength has beauty in its own right and you must be strong to turn society around and effect essential changes that are well overdue.

IN THE NAME OF FASHION

The process of change has already begun and even in small measure it is a step in the right direction. To their credit the French government has stepped in to protect impressionable young girls and women from risking their lives to attain the 'perfect' body. In a groundbreaking bill they intend to make it illegal to publish images on websites and place ads in magazines and other media which promote 'extreme thinness.'

With fines of $70,000 and a possible three year jail sentence it is an effort to stop pro-anorexic websites that give young women advice on how to manipulate doctors and to get by on one apple a day or a few lettuce leaves. With 30,000 to 40,000 anorexics in France, most of whom are women, it's a matter of urgency. The French fashion industry has agreed to sign a charter to promote a healthier body image.

This is an essential move since a survey there concluded that most French women chose as their ideal beauty an image of a fourteen year old girl. Despite claims that French women don't get fat by indulging in long walks and a restricted healthy diet, it's more likely their lean figures are achieved by puffing away on cigarettes at Parisian cafes, limiting food intake and drinking copious cups of strong coffee.

France has by far the highest proportion of clinically underweight women in Europe but only half of them actually think they are too thin according to a new study. The study also shows that what people consider to be an ideal weight in France is lower than in other countries. So the researchers conclude that, 'if a French person who feels fat were to go to the United States, which has a much higher level of obesity, they probably wouldn't feel fat anymore.'

I beg to differ. We're talking about a state of mind here. The French person would probably think the American was massive and run back to their hotel room and go without lunch so that they wouldn't turn out that way. What we have here is a frail deer that wandered out of the forest and ended up in an elephant park. Not for a moment do they feel better but rather very much threatened. It's all about species.

Gender also comes into it. In Western Europe men tip the scales as overweight in every country except France and the Netherlands. By contrast women are considered heavy in only three countries – Greece, Britain and Portugal. Men and women perceive their weight in different ways. Men have a hard time when they're underweight but don't seem to have much of a problem when they're overweight. Probably because men are historically the 'protectors' and don't like to be seen as puny or weak. Women who are underweight don't devalue it but when they pack on the pounds they freak out. So for men weight is perceived as strength while women consider it unwanted and unsightly, perhaps a throwback to earlier times when they were meek and needed protection.

The focus on being 'thin' is most extreme in the modeling world where gaunt young women strut their stuff. The Spanish have already instigated measures to banish models with a body mass index of less than eighteen from the runway. Meanwhile the mayor of Milan was shot down in flames when she insisted something be done in Italy by the head of the national chamber of fashion. He claimed models were healthy and voluptuous but his measure must have been a stick insect.

Under pressure, the Italian government signed a manifesto requiring that models present a doctor's certificate declaring them free from eating disorders before they could model in Milan. However models at the fashion week said no one asked for any proof and they were as thin as ever. The Italians should know better for, unlike the French, they traditionally favor voluptuous women.

The heiress to the Versace Empire, Allegra Versace, is a tragic example of how fashion can spin out of control. The young woman has fought an ongoing battle with anorexia and illustrates how the slimming disease has become 'the dark secret of the fashion world'. An Italian model named Ilaria died of anorexia at 27 years of age, her Saturn return, after struggling with the illness for ten years. She weighed just seventy pounds at the time of her death, the same as Allegra at her worst. About half of the sufferers of anorexia recover within four years, one quarter improve and one quarter remains severely underweight. After ten years recovery is rare and 3% die within that time, half of them by suicide. What an unnecessary tragedy and a terrible waste of beautiful souls.

In some South American countries modeling agencies are now demanding models prove their health with medical certificates but again how efficiently is this policed? This follows the death of several top models from anorexia, including the Brazilian beauty Ana Carolina Reston in 2006. Ana died of kidney failure at twenty one, after living on a diet of tomatoes and apples. She was a model for Armani, but to their credit they called her agency after she did a photo shoot for their catalogue and advised them that she was too thin. Luis Ramsel was a model from Uruguay who died minutes after stepping off the catwalk. She had barely survived on a diet of lettuce leaves and diet soda.

It has been claimed that many South American contestants in beauty pageants have been manufactured since birth. Venezuela has won more global competitions that any other country and has many natural beauties. However it is common practice to alter your features there, and as one young woman said, 'breast surgery is normal just like streaking your hair.' Even more disturbing is the Miss Plastic Surgery beauty contest held in China, where plastic surgery is a billion dollar business and the fastest growing one. The only criteria for entering is that you must prove that your beauty is *man-made*. Sigh.

The proposed French bill had mixed reactions. The head of the French Federation of Couture strongly disapproved. A spokesman for Chanel stated, 'the fashion industry is not responsible for anorexia. Fashion is a reflection of changes in society. It is not the cause. People shouldn't try to turn the issue into a fashion world drama.' *But it is.* On the plus side, Armani said 'I never liked thin girls and never made them go out on the catwalk.' Which is just as well because a casting director at one French agency said that during Fashion Week, 'the models were so thin. It's really scary, like a concentration camp.' I thought the war was over and if not it should be before we kill off all our young girls.

It's no wonder we still battle with comments like these from one top French designer. 'What I really don't like was that certain fashion sizes were made bigger. What I created was fashion for slim, slender people.' According to this philosophy, the rest of us, the majority in fact, are so unworthy we can go hang out in a potato sack for the rest of our lives. It's time the fashion world woke up to itself. It is setting a dreadful example and impossible standards. It's been claimed that a number of gay designers tailor their clothes for an androgynous or slight, male figure rather than for a full figured woman but the problem goes much deeper. Designers insist on their freedom as creators. 'Fashion must be excessive,' Nathalie, the daughter of designer Sonia Rykiel, said. 'The woman on the catwalk represents the artistic vision of the creators. Woman on the street must adapt it to their own bodies.'

No amount of adaptation is going to solve this issue. Most people can't afford to buy one piece of designer clobber, let alone the three it would take to make one dress for the rest of us. And why should we have to? As one lady I met in the changing room the other day said, 'Big people deserve to look good too.' Amen. The art of design is not restrictive and size is immaterial when it comes to creative genius.

When I was a teenager I was forced to make my own clothes because nothing ever fit. It served me well because later in life I opened my own boutique in Bali. My clothes sold well and I ended up doing successful fashion shows at several large resorts and hotels. Restricted to Indonesian models, my fashions started off as smaller sizes. It was easy enough preening the models and dressing them up but I wanted more. So I designed for real women and decided to use the guests at the hotel as my models. Selecting a group of women around the pool, I dressed each one individually according to their unique shape and size.

It was more challenging than using clothes hanger models but infinitely more satisfying. The women were thrilled to show off their style and grace and my sales soared. I even had one classy European gent come up after one show and say, 'This is better than any show I've seen in Milan or Paris!' It's all in the presentation and the love.

The word 'vogue' derives from the French word to be stylish and in fashion. As I flicked through several issues of Vogue magazine at the hairdresser I was horrified. They appeared to have plucked the most emaciated females from all corners of the globe and offered them up as the jewels of fashion. They were all tall and angular, pale and gaunt, hollow eyed and vacant, and nothing I ever wanted to be. With such distorted images of the female form it is encouraging to see that the magazine is bowing to pressure, publishing a Vogue Annual Shape edition which comes out in April. So all us chubbies, shorties, mums and 'normals' can come out of the closet once a year and with any luck might be actually able to buy something to fill it. Maybe.

Inside the Vogue shape edition we find superb photos of the plus size model Crystal Renn. A stunning curvaceous woman, or at least she was. She looked like the goddess Venus incarnate until I spotted her in a recent magazine. She had shed a lot of weight and lost her original spark. Why would one of the highest paid plus size models in the world succumb to pressure to alter her fabulous looks and become ordinary?

The words 'vogued' or 'voguing' mean 'to dance while striking a rigid, stylized poses evocative of fashion models doing fashion shoots.' Now rigid I can see and stylized yes. But dancing, no, unless we are talking about those darling ballerinas who flit across the stage in gossamer tulle and satin pumps mincing about to Swan Lake. Nothing like the ample opera singers who thump about in their flatties and make a lot of noise. So much so they need to be removed from the stage.

If the critical review on opera singers was not enough we can now be suitably outraged, and appropriately lots of people are, about the recent attack on a lovely ballerina and her partner. A high profile ballet critic caustically wrote that the New York City Ballet's principal dancer was too fat and looked 'like she'd eaten one sugar plum too many to play the Sugar Plum Fairy while her partner seems to have been sampling half the sweet realm.' A photo of the two performers shows a sublimely slim and beautiful couple, so to retaliate I demand to see what the scathing critic looks like on the stage in tights. The ballet they were performing was The Nutcracker, appropriate in so many ways.

It's all too ridiculous. We love people because they have a special essence, a quality that shines from every pore of their body. Beauty comes in many varied packages and that's what keeps it interesting and beguiling. When persons in the spotlight change or conform to a stereotype they take away the essence that attracted us in the first place. Look what happened to Jennifer Grey from Dirty Dancing. She just changed the shape of her nose and that was enough to end her career.

We are not dolls, we are people. Each one of us is attractive in our right. Included in the Vogue shape edition were interviews with lovely Queen Latifah and Keely Shaye Smith. Keely was a former soap opera star and is wife to the suave Pierce Brosnan. She was captured on film while she was on holiday wearing a bikini over her ample curves. It provoked derisive comments among the vacuous of mind. I applaud her for stating that she 'was proud of her Rubenesque figure', while her husband Pierce said that he 'loved his wife's curves and thought she was stunning.' These are the type of people who will change the world.

When the spokesmen for Chanel stated that fashion had no bearing on anorexia, he was sorely out of touch. Once again it begs the question, 'Why do women have to torture themselves to reduce their body size so they can look like an anorexic model who is about to keel over from hunger, do a back flip off the runway in her killer shoes and tumble straight into a spiritual vacuum and worse still, the lap of the blessed designer. Does anyone in the fashion world get it or even care, or are they desperate to save on the cost of material?

In that parallel universe we call fashion, the clothes bear little or no resemblance to reality. It's not artistic grandeur to design for an unreal shapeless form but a gross act of VANITY. On your part. You are not serving society or adding anything very positive to the *real* world. Instead you are pandering to your own ego while destroying ours. You make women feel less than they are because they can't measure up to some impossible standard that is sorely out of reach.

Just take a look at many of the designers taking a bow at the end of a fashion show. Most look short and sheepish because deep down they know that they, or their sisters or mothers, could never fit into their clothes. Many don't have the slightest idea of how a real woman looks and even less desire to discover it, or to work with it. So designers, rather than try to change us to conform to your perception of idealized beauty dress *us* to be the ideal beauty. Normal and yes, even big women deserve to look good. We must break free from this travesty of so called fashion for there is more to life than this. There is true style.

A STATE OF GRACE

The show 'How to Look Good Naked' captured extraordinary ratings for Lifetime television in the US when it was first introduced. In each episode, the exuberant Carson Kressley takes two women who are suffering from poor self esteem and deals them a harsh reality check. They strip down to their underwear and look into a mirror to see their real selves. Their reluctance to take a look is tragic.

Why? Because they don't see the image of beauty that has been fed to us over a lifetime looking back at them. They're not Cinderella with a pink satin ribbon in her hair, plastic Barbie in seven inch stilettos, a stunning Victoria Secret's model or a size zero starlet in a vintage Dior frock. No, what they see is themselves and it repulses them. What have we done to create such a massive meltdown in our people? These women are so depressed by the reflection of themselves that some refuse to get out of bed in the morning or to leave the house. Their husbands still love them as do their children but they do not love who they are, now or if ever.

When they are asked to place themselves in a line up of women according to their size most get it wrong because they believe they are much larger than they actually are. As their perception alters and their confidence builds they take the plunge and allow themselves to be photographed in the nude. What an incredible leap of faith. The photo is then splashed across a huge billboard in the center of the city.

Shock, horror. The women are overwhelmed and cry bitter tears as they listen to the comments of people passing by. 'That's what real beauty is,' one astute man says, adding, 'if it wasn't for her wedding ring I'd ask her out.' Another says 'She's hot,' while another comments on 'how sexy is she,' or 'that's called keeping it real.'

People are not as shallow as we make them out to be. Most get it. They understand that beauty truly does emanate from within to reflect on the outside. It's a state of being and is all about energy. Anyone with positive energy attracts others but it's hard when you don't match the 'ideal' beauty to continue to radiate self confidence. Slowly it gets eroded away until we feel empty and only the hardiest person retains their original spark. Fortunately it can be brought back. In just three short days the women's self image is turned around. Positive comments, a little sprucing up and an ego boost erases years of degradation.

Never underestimate how damaging our society is and how traumatic these issues are. Two stories serve to remind us. The first is of a large lady who lives in a country town in Australia. She is well known in the community but one day when she fell over nobody came to her aid. It took her some time to get on her feet and her spirit shrunk from the shame. Worn down from the continual humiliation, this woman refused to get out of bed in the end. Frustrating years of diets, grim forecasts by doctors, failed weight support groups and an array of diet aids and pills led not to weight loss but rather to loss of self.

Then came the terrible fate of an Indonesian lass, a cousin of a friend of mine in Jakarta. The girl was ribbed at school for being fat even though she was only slightly plump and carried very little excess flesh. The rest of the girls were reed thin and gave her a hard time. Defeated she succumbed to pressure and stopped eating while binging on diet pills and laxatives. One day she went to the toilet at a restaurant and her insides fell out, literally. She died a tragic, horrible death.

These are horrendous stories and there are many more. It's the most terrible tragedy that society is slowly killing its own kind. Ironically it's doing it under the guise of trying to save them. It claims to care about their plight yet it heaps more and more pressure on an overloaded soul to conform to an unrealistic standard, until they break. With our current obsession with body shape we pay a hefty price because we have overlooked the most important part of our selves, the part that carries the most weight ... our soul. With such a heavy burden, it suffers. No amount of looking in the mirror will heal our spirit, yet reflect we must if we are to finally get it right.

I was in Bali during the time of the horrific bombings when many lives were lost. It was a shocking time and I took time out to heal back in Australia. Realizing that it could have been me, I understood just how lucky I was to be alive, both at that time and after my brain surgery. One day when I was sitting on my balcony reflecting on the fragility of life an angelic voice whispered in my ear. I was hoping to hear words that were profound as they were comforting but instead I was given these simple words, *'Did you eat enough ice cream?'* At first I thought I was hallucinating, imagining a dying man's last wish.

Notice how a dying man's last wish is food related. They don't ask the condemned man on Death Row which book he wants to read or TV program to watch, or game of sport, or even to have sex for the last time. No, the final request is, 'What do you want for your last meal?' Life's ultimate pleasure becomes its last. Back to the ice cream. After giving much thought to the words, 'Did you eat enough ice cream?' it slowly began to sink in. Simply put it meant, 'Did you enjoy your life?' Despite everything life offered you, in spite of all the challenges and the obstacles you had to face, did you have a good time?

That's when I finally got it. When I truly understood. Life is a celebration. It should be grabbed with both hands and embraced and squeezed hard until the last drop of experience, angst and happiness is extracted from it. Yes, it can be hard at times when you are forced to climb that mountain and stumble over the rocks but when you discover the diamonds it will be worth it. And the view at the top is magnificent.

Never let anyone tell you can't do it, whatever *it* may be, or that you don't deserve to succeed or to enjoy your life. Don't let them try to convince you that you're too fat, too old, too inept or not good enough. **If someone puts you down, lift them up.** They need help and you're the better person. You just have to believe it. You will believe it when you achieve 'your state of grace'. Your inner bliss.

Exactly how does one achieve a state of grace? That ideal state when mind, body and soul are in perfect harmony. Acceptance. It's that simple. You have to accept yourself, warts and all. You must be proud of who you are and what you were born to achieve. In spite of all the pressure to change or to conform, you must remain true to yourself. You are perfect as you were intended to be but first you must believe it.

Harmony will occur when you get in touch with your Higher self. Once you have reconnected you will be at peace. Your outer shell, your outward appearance, is not determined by diet or weight or hair color but rather by attitude. It reflects the state of your being and the essence you bring to the world. So now take a few minutes and find a quiet space where you can be alone. Get comfortable and then close your eyes. Take a few deep breaths and center yourself. Slowly in your mind's eye form a picture of your true self. THE REAL YOU. Many people don't have a clue of who they are because they have always been reminded of who they aren't.

Now see the real you. Not the Disney version with an impossible waistline and birds chirping as they serenade you and squirrels running at your feet, and not the Vogue edition that would shrink or elongate you into a stylized caricature. Or the negative image of yourself that has been built up over the years as you have been compared with some impossible ideal. Instead see who you are truly meant to be as part of your family, with your own distinctive DNA and racial heritage, your astrological pattern and your unique sense of self. THAT IS THE REAL YOU.

Breathe deeply and let go of any anger, resentment or sorrow that you may feel at being discriminated against or not recognized for who you are. I understand those emotions but be careful that you don't shoot yourself in the foot along the way. You are harming yourself more than you are hurting anyone else by letting negative conditioning win.

No matter the source of your pain, release it. A toxic parent will find something else to complain about if weight ceases to become an issue and a magazine will look for the next star they can shoot down in flames. The doctor will go on to the next patient and forget you were there and true friends will love you anyway. Only invite goodness into your life and positive caring people. You do have a choice. It's in your power to direct the film of your life and to choose its cast of characters. You can opt for a happy ending, or a sad, destructive, painful one.

Is the picture you see of yourself a true reflection of who you are today? If you do not match the image in your mind's eye of a healthy, happy soul then decide on a positive change. Manifest the optimum you. Treat yourself well. If you eat with moderation, intelligence and intent, food will serve you well. You're much smarter than society gives you credit for, so be your own judge and decide what is right for you. But also be compassionate and caring. You are doing the best you can.

Your body is your temple, so treasure it. In turn it will ensure that you are looked after and so remain healthy. Take every opportunity to rejoice in life even though it may seem at times there is little worth celebrating. Find your bliss, the magic of the moment and relish the experience. It's life at its best and you deserve the best.

One New Year's Eve I was alone in my apartment. I could have wallowed in my loneliness but instead I decided to toast my freedom and independence. Not one for champagne, I filled my finest crystal goblet with apple juice. Just before midnight, I dragged a chair onto my balcony and stood on it. Balancing myself precariously I toasted in the New Year as I watched the fireworks explode in the distance over Sydney Harbor, wishing myself a fabulous year to come.

It was my own private celebration of life. Remember if you don't believe you deserve the best no one else will. I recall dating a gorgeous man once who had always relied on his looks. He was spoiled and there was never a shortage of people prepared to pay to be with him. I noticed whenever we ate at a fancy restaurant he always ordered the most expensive dish on the menu while I chose the cheapest. It was never a question of money. It was just that he believed he warranted the best while subconsciously I devalued myself.

I learnt much from that man. Without meaning to he taught me how to appreciate myself. It took a long time to reprogram my thinking. Growing up I had felt unworthy at times but once I became an adult it was entirely up to me. So I made the conscious choice to realize my worth and spoil myself. Enjoy the best life has to offer. You deserve it.

BEAUTY IS ONLY SKIN DEEP

Historically if we look at people who have left their mark upon the world, very few did so because of their beauty. In fact, beauty at best is transient and often leads to a sad end. Movie stars were lauded for their looks but it did them no good in the long run when faced with the harsh realities of life. Vivacious redhead Rita Hayworth was cut down by Alzheimer's disease while stunning Vivien Leigh of Gone With the Wind fame succumbed to mental illness. The screen goddess Marilyn Monroe died either by suicide or by foul play. Luscious Elizabeth Taylor battled many illnesses and a string of husbands to emerge stronger, and her beauty is mirrored in her lifelong struggle.

Beauty can afford an easy ticket through life for some but vanity catches up with them in the end. The infamous queen of France, Marie Antoinette, had no concern for the hardship of her people and preferred to revel in the finer things in life. A self absorbed Scorpio she is attributed with the classic quote, 'Let them eat cake,' when her people had no bread to eat and were starving and on the brink of a revolution.

Her philosophy did not win favor and Marie met an unhappy end at the guillotine. Another beauty who had her head chopped off, although her executioner used an axe, was Ann Boleyn of England. She used her beauty to capture King Henry 8th but he soon tired of it and went on to marry the plainer Jane Seymour who bore him a son. Jane died soon after but she must have had more substance because, of all his wives, the king chose to be buried beside her in Windsor Cathedral.

The Egyptian queen Cleopatra was portrayed as a wanton temptress whose beauty changed the fate of the Roman Empire. She was accused of being a sorceress and all sorts of evil doings. After the deaths of her two lovers, Julius Caesar and Marc Anthony, and her capture, she reputedly put an end to her own life by placing an asp to her bosom and letting it do its worst. This was one queen who was highly dramatic till the end.

Mata Hari used her allure to entice men in high position to spill their secrets and became one of the most infamous spies of all time. A Dutch woman with an active imagination, she pretended to be a high caste Hindu Javanese princess and became an exotic dancer who slept with many high ranking military officers, politicians and the Crown Prince of Germany. It did her no good because she still met a sticky end. A message intercepted by the French during World War 2, which may have been planted by the Germans, was enough to convict her of being a spy. She was executed by a French firing squad at the age of forty one. True to her sign, Leo, she went out with a flourish. To some accounts in a well designed suit and blowing a kiss at her executioners.

The peerless beauty of Helen was enough to tear the ancient kingdom of Troy apart, evidence that it's not such a good thing to be so gorgeous that men fall at your feet and launch a thousand ships to fetch you back. It's understandable why veils came into fashion and why sultry Salome was kept under wraps with all her whirling paraphernalia and chiffon scarves.

Till today beauty is as fickle as it is temperamental. Supermodel Naomi Campbell is renowned for her hissy fits of rage and I wouldn't want to cross Angelina Jolie in any way or admit to my lust for Brad. On a recent program that showed charming society debutantes, we were introduced to lovely lasses with names like Tamsen, Dympna and Perfidia. Apparently these girls had it 'all'. *All* meaning fancy homes, expensive cars and designer handbags and shoes. That's it? Even the dimmest beauty pageant contestant knows, 'What about World Peace?'

This sort of mentality promotes nothing but an obsession with superficial appearance and materialistic gain. Even though, 'one can never be too thin or too rich', you can definitely be too shallow, vain, inane, vacant and artificial. Are these the role models we want our children to aspire to? If this is the future of our world then we're in big trouble. The people who left their mark on history were as

171

distinctive and varied in their looks as they were distinguished in their achievements or diabolical in their intentions.

They each impacted on us in their own way. Italian dictator Mussolini was stubby and Napoleon compensated for his short stature by building empires. Artist Toulouse Lautrec was crippled from birth, his body stunted but not his spirit. Most nights he frequented the Moulin Rouge and immortalized its sumptuous dancers in his paintings. Winston Churchill, Nikita Khrushchev, Golda Meir and Mao Tse Tung were portly while Abraham Lincoln towered over others. With their eccentric looks Einstein and Mozart are instantly recognizable, Yoko Ono and Bob Marley developed their own unique style, Joseph Stalin, Che Guevara and Fidel Castro were fierce, Woody Allen and Twiggy are slight. Helen Keller was deaf, dumb and blind and look what she managed to achieve. Now there's true inspiration.

The following is a list of people who inspired mankind while others provoked us into action. They have been listed astrologically so they can encourage others of their sign to achieve their own potential or conversely never to step out of line. Good or bad, they each impacted on the world as we know it, in their own unique significant way. As you can see from the list, beauty had very little to do with it.

ARIES

Strong willed and egotistical, the ram endows us with a diverse but dynamic mix. Comedian Charlie Chaplin, Russian president Nikita Khrushchev, singer Billie Holiday, the artist Goya, the writers Samuel Becket, Emile Zola and Joseph Pulitzer, the poet William Wordsworth, Kofi Annan, the former UN Secretary General, the composer Bach, and the horniest ram of all, Playboy's Hugh Hefner.

TAURUS

The strong feminine energy of Taurus gives us the powerful female leaders Queen Elizabeth II of England and Catherine the Great of Russia. Then there was Florence Nightingale, the scientist Marconi, the voice of Barbara Streisand, the style of Liberace, the depth of psychoanalyst Sigmund Freud and the genius of artist, inventor and mathematician Leonardo da Vinci.

GEMINI

Another strong bunch, each with attributes that make them unique. US president John F. Kennedy, writer Salman Rushdie, billionaire Donald Trump, Che Guevara and Queen Victoria are all forces to be reckoned with. Then comes the creative spirit of architect Frank Lloyd Wright, dancer Isadora Duncan, artists Gaugin and Constable, the composers Wagner and Cole Porter and singers Bob Dylan and Judy Garland.

CANCER

Men of vision were the Greek explorer Alexander the Great, Roman Emperor Julius Caesar and spiritual leaders the Dalai Lama and Nelson Mandela. Others who left their mark on history were King Henry the Eighth, the writer Ernest Hemingway, Nelson Rockefeller, the sensitive Princess Diana and determined Helen Keller. Artists include Rembrandt and Degas, and designers Armani, Cardin and Oscar de la Renta.

LEO

As expected with the lion that roars and likes to make his presence felt, we have a rather strong minded lot. They include Bill Clinton, Fidel Castro, Napoleon Bonaparte, Zapata the Mexican revolutionary and the Italian Fascist dictator Benito Mussolini. Then there was the adventurous aviator Amelia Earheart, Neil Armstrong the first man to step foot on the Moon and the spy Mata Hari. Creatively they are rather eccentric like artist Andy Warhol and Harry Potter's J K Rowling.

VIRGO

This pristine sign ranges in extremes from the saint-like Mother Teresa to the brutal Ivan the Terrible. Somewhere in between are

Louis 14th, the Sun King of France, magician David Copperfield, psychologists Dr. Joyce Brothers and Dr. Phil who like to probe into the inner sanctum of your mind and dish out advice on how to clean up your act, Yassar Arafat, Twiggy, golfer Arnold Palmer, conductor Leonard Bernstein, the great Michael Jackson and my personal favorite Mickey Mouse.

LIBRA

A sign of peace and accord, it is not surprising that notable Librans include Alfred Nobel, founder of the Nobel Prize, pacifist Mahatma Ghandi, humanitarian Bob Geldorf, the inspired John Lennon, writers Arthur Miller and Doris Lessing, Eleanor Roosevelt, Margaret Thatcher, composer Verdi and the spiritualists Annie Bessant and the mysterious master of the occult Aleister Crowley.

SCORPIO

As expected the scorpion gathers a more eclectic mix with a dark edge. Pablo Picasso the artist with his wild deranged imagination, French Queen Marie Antoinette, Leo Trotsky, Goebbels, the Nazi officer and Grace Slick. On the brighter side of dark hoping to enlighten the world are Carl Sagan the scientist, Indira Ghandi, the philosopher Voltaire, the inspirational Martin Luther King and billionaire Bill Gates.

SAGITTARIUS

Aiming to spread their wisdom across the world are the British wartime Prime Minister Winston Churchill, Indian mystic Sai Baba, American billionaire John Paul Getty, anthropologist Margaret Mead, writers Jane Austin and Mark Twain, the composer Ludwig Beethoven, the artist Toulouse Lautrec and directors Woody Allen and Stephen Spielberg.

CAPRICORN

Concerned with business and making money are wealthy Howard Hughes and Conrad Hilton, followed by the determined mix of boxer

Muhamed Ali, science fiction writer Isaac Asimov, the Russian leader Joseph Stalin and Chinese leader Mao Tse Tung, artist Matisse, scientist Isaac Newton and cosmetic queens Elizabeth Arden and Helena Rubinstein. To add a spiritual touch to this materialistic sign are the mystic Nostradamus and present day psychic Jeanne Dixon.

AQUARIUS

An intellectual air sign that thinks outside the box, it includes many acclaimed writers and poets. Sir Francis Bacon, Robert Burns, Virginia Woolf, Germaine Greer, Charles Dickens, Chekov and Lord Byron, to name a few. Also the composers Mozart and Schubert, the US presidents Abraham Lincoln and Franklin D Roosevelt, the military general Douglas Macarthur, the evolutionist Charles Darwin, Christian Dior, Bob Marley, Yoko Ono, Babe Ruth and Frederico Fellini.

PISCES

Pisces can be a brilliant sign, with a deeply imaginative mind. Included among its ranks are nuclear physicist and genius Albert Einstein, the children's writer Dr. Seuss, the African explorer David Livingstone, US president George Washington, the media mogul Rupert Murdoch, the eccentric Gloria Vanderbilt, writer Victor Hugo and Yuri Gagarin, the Russian astronaut and first person into space.

These are some of the people who have left their mark upon society. *In the end it didn't matter their shape because they helped shape our world.* They were far less interested in their own beauty but rather in what they could create to make the world more beautiful. These are the people we truly remember … the artists, the writers, composers, statesmen, empire builders, the adventurers, the scientists, the healers and the visionaries. Even those who brought negative energy impacted on us. They ultimately made us better people by reminding us of our principles and the creed we live by. They forced us to take a deeper look and re-evaluate and in the end made us stand up and fight for what we believed to be right. And so we took a closer step towards the light.

BEAUTY IS IN
THE EYE OF THE BEHOLDER

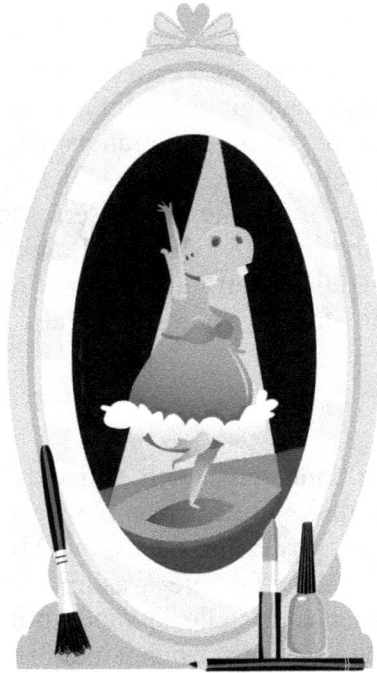

Did you read about the recent discovery of a statue, believed to be the oldest one on earth? If not, here it is in a nutshell.

May 2009. 'BERLIN - A 35,000-year-old ivory carving of a busty woman found in a German cave was unveiled last week by archaeologists who believe it to be the oldest known sculpture of the human form. Fragments found in a German cave depict a woman with a swollen belly, wide-set thighs and large, protruding breasts.'

'It's very sexually charged,' said the university archaeologist who discovered the figure. 'The discovery suggests that humans who are believed to have come to Europe 40,000 years ago had the intelligence to create symbols and think abstractly like the modern human. It's one hundred percent certain that 40,000 years ago in Swabia (where!) we're dealing with people just like you and me.'

Whoa, stop there! Does anyone apart from me see the fat fly in the ointment? We're talking about 40,000 years ago, the first people to tread upon European soil and we're talking about fatties. *'People just like you and me'*. Women with large bellies, pear shaped thighs and big breasts. These people couldn't pin their bulk on Herr Fritz's Wiener sausages or Frau Linzel's hazelnut torte, so what's going on?

Were the Swabians a hoggish race and if so what did they have to pig out on? A hearty soup of reed grasses or a pungent mix of bat droppings and herbs? Or could it possibly be this scandalous truth. *That people were just born like that.* A Teutonic race who were big boned and large. Could I be radical enough to suggest that there is no other feasible explanation for their size except to say that's how they were created, and that's how they were intended? Voluptuous and grand.

Now if you're cynical and hard headed, refusing to believe that some of us were just meant to be big, let's consider another hypothesis. Let's say the Swabians were a midget race with great expectations. Was there one errant Swabian lady who let her appetite run away with her? Did she gorge herself on mammoth bones when no one else was looking or indulge in one too many brontosaurus burgers? Did she not join the rest of the clan for their daily mountain hike looking for stray yaks or refuse to run rings around the Paleolithic stone circle?

If in fact she was an aberrant Swabian, the only large lady in the pack, then why did the tribe choose to immortalize her? Why was *she* chosen as the epitome of beauty, the one they idolized enough to painstakingly carve her out of ivory to capture her likeness forever? Could it be that back then, big was beautiful?

There are a number of Stone Age carvings that reinforce this notion. Consider the famous Venus statues that date back to early times. These rock carvings depict a woman with exaggerated curves and are considered to be fertility symbols. I think they were the first 'pin ups', a form of beauty that people aspired to be like or ones that encapsulated their concept of the ideal human form. The first time I saw an image of the Venus of Willendorf, the most famous of these Venus statues, was in high school art class. As I looked at my gangly, flat-chested schoolmates there came a bitter blow. Only the Venus and I shared ponderous breasts. She may have been a goddess in her time but I felt less like one and more like the clump of stone she was carved from.

I wanted to be svelte and angular like my classmates. So to compensate I grew my hair long and cast all images of portly stone goddesses from my mind. I was left with the cruel realization that I was born out of time. At the wrong time and in the wrong place. Why wasn't I born at the time of Rubens or Titian? These artists recognized a fabulous woman when they saw one. I would have settled for the ancient Greeks who knew the value of a good set of curves. Even the French once had an eye for a shapely lass but now they have settled for thin waifs with wispy voices. Long gone is the time of Boucher, Matisse and Courbet. Picasso portrayed strange rounded women in his paintings but he was a rampant Spaniard so it doesn't count.

Like everything else in society our concept of beauty changes. That's what stops us from getting stale. Trends come and go. As Heidi Klum would say, 'One day you're in, the next you're out.' There are skinny, lean years and those of abundance and curves and if you're really lucky you may match your era. Fortunately long gone is the time of corsets and lace up bustiers that sucked the life force out of you or times of genteel aristocracy when people wore white powder caked onto their faces and had all sorts of dubious life forms crawling through their bouffant wigs! More dead than alive, no wonder it was difficult to breathe. No wonder they needed leeches to get the blood flowing.

Nor is it the 1920's when the Charleston prevailed, and dancing flappers were not allowed to flap. One ad that I uncovered from that era extolled the virtues of swallowing a tape worm to shed those unwanted pounds. The worm if well trained would eat away at your insides and get fat in your place. It could also kill you in the end. 'Eat! Eat! Eat! & Always Stay Thin.' The ad promised. 'FAT, THE ENEMY banished! How? With Sanitized Tape Worms. Jar Packed. Easy to Swallow. No Ill Effects. Friends for a Fat Form.' I guess if you were fat in those days you might need a friend. It's a shame if the only one you could muster was a worm in a jar. One that would devour your innards and keep a smile on its face. Oh, the things we do in the name of 'beauty'.

So as the worm turns, times change. Curvy came back into vogue after the grey days of the depression and the dismal darkness of the war with a trail of stunning movie stars. Sultry Ava Gardner was a size 14 and all woman, voluptuous Jayne Mansfield and Jane Russell could have done some major damage with their killer breasts, Rita Hayworth was gorgeous when she shimmied in Gilda and the all time sex goddess Marilyn Monroe was plastered into her dress for US president's JFK's birthday ball, showing off her magnificent curves.

Then something happened. Uranus shifted gears. Movies became insipid or violent instead of inspiring and romantic. Glamour was gone and in its place were action movies with robotic stars, as android heroes blasted away the world annihilating any last vestige of sophistication and charm with it. Androgynous was all the vogue and the line that separated female from male was clouded. Fashion mirrored the trend.

Actresses with any femininity starved themselves to meet some perverted ideal not having the strength, courage or numbers to create their own. Further driven to lose their identity, some decided to reinvent themselves. By transplanting butt fat into their cheeks, injecting toxic poisons around their eyes, sucking their souls out from their stomachs and stringing up their faces to look like a trussed up turkey ready for the Sunday roast, they committed a horrid act of self destruction.

I understand that people in the public eye need to maintain a certain level of attractiveness but when that is carried out to the extreme, when they are more android than human, more plastic than elastic, I protest. We idolized them and put them up there on a pedestal in the first place so by presenting this fractured concept of beauty they do us no favors nor our children who will go on to emulate them. The saying 'beauty is only skin deep' is fine but when our society implies that fat blocks that expression of beauty, I take offence. So should you.

Ask me who I think is the most beautiful woman of all time and you would be surprised with my answer. Recently I watched a program on the National Geographic channel which opened my eyes to another reality. As a person who considers herself in tune with the realm of the spiritual, I was excited to discover a topic that had previously eluded me. The program was titled 'Sleeping Beauties' and told of a group of canonized Catholic saints called 'The Indestructibles.'

The reason they are considered 'indestructible' is because when they were dug up after burial, the saints' bodies were found to have remained intact centuries after their death. Remarkable. Their skin looks perfect and their bodies remain lifelike, moist and flexible. Even more amazingly some perspired and their blood still flowed! There is no feasible explanation as to why their bodies did not decay into dust.

In other cases where bodies are preserved there were mitigating factors such as death in dry hot sand or lava, or in sealed chambers with no air or moisture. Others like the ancient Egyptians had been mummified to preserve their bodies. This was not the case with the saints. What also separated them was their spiritual state at the moment of death. In one catacomb under a church in Germany were images of the shriveled remains of the dead. One man's look of horror as he fell to his death, another a distraught woman and her child who lost their lives in tragic circumstances. Their death state mirrors their distress.

With the saints, their faces told another story. They all looked remarkably serene, accepting their passage onto another plane. In some the body was enveloped by the sweet scent of roses that endured for decades after they were excavated from their tombs. The fact that their faces still beamed calm and bright was miraculous. Then came the most beautiful of all. The Sleeping beauty, asleep in her glass casket.

St Bernadette. The young girl from the French village of Lourdes who had visions of a beautiful lady standing amongst the bushes. The girl who purportedly received messages from the virgin mother and inspired Lourdes with its legion of pilgrims who come seeking a miracle cure from its healing spring. St Bernadette, a young woman who endured a life of crippling sickness, died in 1879 at the age of 35.

Over one hundred years later gazing at her body exhumed from her grave I have never seen such a vision of beauty. I am not a religious person but gazing upon that woman is a spiritual revelation. In her death state St. Bernadette is supremely beautiful. She is all at once serene, accepting and appears to be staring into the eyes of the divine. She is just as stunningly beautiful in death as she was in life. Her beauty did not disappear with death but rather it was enhanced.

I would be remiss not to mention another of the indestructible saints. A portly, happy woman she was a nun who devoted her life to creating missions across the world for displaced children. In her death state she looks sweet of heart and round of body. The look on her face is sheer bliss. What is even more remarkable is this fact. Centuries later, SHE WEIGHS EXACTLY THE SAME DEAD AS SHE DID WHEN SHE WAS ALIVE. Even after she passed away she couldn't lose any weight because that was the form her body was meant to be. Mind you, not for a moment do I believe that she ever tried. She was far too busy with her mission, following her calling and far too content with life.

LIVING OFF THE FAT
OF THE LAND

Let's take a moment. Make yourself a nice cup of herbal tea, flop into your favorite recliner and put your feet up. Now let's take the opportunity to 'chew the fat'. Let's discuss what's on our minds. Are you as disgusted as I am with the current trend of 'fat bashing?' Are you as outraged as I am that fat is being blamed for every affliction known to mankind? Angered by the insinuation that the broader of our species are causing the demise of the modern world as we know it.

Now take another bite of your diet cookie and think it over. One slap in the face after another. 'You've got no self control, you're an inert slob, you take up too much room and you're placing stress on the medical system because it's collapsing under the weight of your clotted arteries.' Oh, sigh. Every day there's another report in the newspaper or accusation splashed across the pages. Another massive blow to the ego.

However when the abuse gets so blatant, one must sit up and take notice. Take the recent report by two British researchers that 'Obesity is killing the planet.' These two brilliant minds from the London School of Hygiene and Tropical Medicine maintain that overweight people are creating a hole in the ozone layer by causing excess greenhouse gas emissions. This is based on a very shaky hypothesis, 'because they eat more than thin people and are more likely to travel by car.' This conclusion is offensive, derisive and highly insulting to every large person in the known universe and I demand an apology on their behalf.

'When it comes to food consumption, moving about in a heavy body is like driving around in a gas guzzler,' the researchers wrote in their study. I suggest these lads don't suggest their theory to an angry hippo, whose stocky legs have been designed to carry its weight. These very limbs will pound these weedy researchers into the ground. After much thought, the gents calculated that a fatter population needs 19 percent more food energy for its requirements. The production of that food requires machinery that emits greenhouse gases, as well as extra transport systems that emit pollution.

Now I hate to quibble but a truck is a truck and a bus is a bus. A train is a train. Twenty fat people, thirty thin ones. Half empty, half full. It's all the same. The bus still trundles around the same old route with enough savvy not to care. The grain train continues down the same tired tracks carrying its heavy load. The researchers continue in the same ridiculous vein, 'a heavier population is dependent on greenhouse gas-emitting cars to help move around its people who have grown too obese to walk.' Call out the tanks! We're talking about half the population who have been erroneously deemed overweight and I don't see them all limping around on canes and walkers to get down to the local mall. My bet is the lean mean researchers will need a cane long before I do.

For their *coup de grace*, the scientists say that the global obesity epidemic needs to be reversed to not only save lives but also to save the environment. I'm deeply offended because I fight hard to save trees not to mention whales. Now I have a novel notion. After lengthy discussion with several lovely slender friends of mine they graciously agreed to sacrifice themselves for a higher good. If they go, I get to stay. So here's my solution. Simple. Cull two thin persons for every fat one and the problem goes away. The two scientists would be the first to go in my book. Now let me share a few comments I found while trawling the internet which sums up how others feel about this study.

'This is absolutely a crazy study. What's wrong with the world is that we are always trying to change it and the idiots who keep on putting out stupid studies that make us feel that there is something wrong with us. What ever happened to living life and just being happy?'

'Do I get carbon credits for being thin?'

'This is too ridiculous for words. First it was CFC's in fridges, then gas guzzling cars followed by too many methane producing cows. Now it's that we're all too fat!'

Let me interject here. The study estimated that each fat person is responsible for about one ton of carbon dioxide emissions each year more than a thin person. That adds up to an extra one billion tons of CO_2 each year in a population of one billion overweight people. Here I must agree. The study definitely provoked a severe case of flatulence in many people, so there *was* an increase of carbon emissions of the more noxious variety. Now if all that methane gas could be harnessed we could save the planet, enjoy ourselves immensely and have a darn good purge in the process! Then channel all that potent energy into the vents of the building where the researchers work and we'll be set for life!

Now one final thought provoking comment. 'All you thin people start your rant! We have moved past speaking negatively about people with alternative lifestyles, minorities and folks that are different than we are but it is still OK to knock fat people. Until then pass the mustard and no I won't steal your place on the plane!' Which brings us to this great brainwave that came out of England's close neighbor Ireland.

'Irish Airline Considering 'Fat Tax'

DUBLIN – Irish budget airline Ryanair is looking at how it can introduce a 'fat tax' after almost a third of travelers voted to penalize obese fellow passengers. (Bravo for the majority of others!) Ryanair says it will now ask travelers how any such charge could be levied. The four options include charging male passengers who weigh over 280 pounds or females over 220 pounds, for every extra pound they weigh. I sense a law suit here. How come men get to take up more space and we have to carry around boobs and butt to boot? It really doesn't matter your sex, one fatty should be allowed to take up as much space as the other regardless of what's going on between their loins!

Another alternative that the brilliant airline has come up with is charging for a second seat if a passenger's waist touches both armrests simultaneously. Oh gosh, just envision the squirming going on in the seats to make sure your bulging midriff doesn't touch the sides. Consider young hostess Colleen skulking up and down the aisles with a ruler to check out where your bits reach or measuring your nether regions. Then cabin attendant Sean whacking you over the head with the life vest, while proclaiming, 'Who's been a naughty girl then,' and refusing to give you any refreshments on your Transatlantic flight even when you paid for them. In advance!

Now I must admit to great embarrassment when I fly a certain budget Asian airline with seatbelts designed to fit miniscule races. I can do the seatbelt up ... just, but in a matter of minutes I feel the onset of a sciatic attack and my toes start to turn a bloodless shade of blue. My cries for help soon bring the tiny hostess scuttling down the aisle, but with her limited grasp of English she has trouble deciphering my pleas. Then with a loud flourish, she yells out loud. 'Ooh, you need seatbelt extender.' I want to strangle myself with the belt at this stage but the desperate looks of other rounded passengers comfort me.

The seatbelt extender was obviously designed for pregnant Russians and is far too big. With no way to be secure in my seat, I pray for a calm flight. The first gust of wind would blow me wildly around the cabin and with any sign of turbulence I would end up in first class where I belong. Hopefully with deluxe size seat belts.

Back to Ryanair. A spokesman for the airline declared proudly, 'These changes, if introduced, might also act as an incentive to some of our very large passengers to lose a little weight.' Imagine it. A line up of passengers in the loo expunging their lunch so they might shed that dreaded last pound to avoid the horrid fat tax. Women dressing as men so they get an extra sixty pound allowance. Lovely Morag at the check in counter announcing over the loudspeaker, 'Paddy hit the scales at ten pounds over and he has to pay the price,' and the whole terminal erupting into thunderous applause. Where does it end? It's ludicrous.

I'm wondering if Paddy brought his lovely girlfriend Kathleen along for the trip and she was a thin wisp of a thing, would he get a rebate? Would the airline staff be up to the task, weighing up both and dividing by two and splitting the difference? Could a desperate fatty grab someone's child and pretend that it was hers, hoping for the sympathy lightweight vote? The possibilities are endless as are the dreadful repercussions.

Now I'm the first to admit that each passenger, no matter their means of transport, deserves their comfort. One disgruntled Aussie sued a US bus company for being jammed against a very large gent for a long road trip. The Aussie came away with a severe injury to his back from being pushed out of shape. This is by no means acceptable. If you are so big that you may cause another person an injury then you must rethink your travel plans and make suitable concessions to avoid doing another person harm. This situation requires careful consideration from passenger and carrier alike and a tenable solution found.

But please do not single out big people. I had a raging argument with a tall, rangy and super opinionated ex Fleet St. Journalist who wrote a health column. As we discussed the issue of weight he got very hot under the collar. The veins in his forehead began to bulge and he started sweating pure venom. 'You can't tell me large people shouldn't be penalized,' he raged, 'for taking up two seats.' There it was again. The assumption that large equaled gross. Not plus size, just gross.

'I'm talking about normal large,' I replied, fixated on a throbbing artery in his neck. I had been trying to make the point that size remains the single worst form of discrimination that exists in our society today but he wasn't having a bar of it. 'I've just booked a trip to the US,' I continued, refusing to concede defeat, 'and for an extra $50 I could have reserved the long seats on the plane, with extra leg room. How come you can be long but not wide? Tell me that's not discrimination.'

Mr. Journalist spluttered in surprise and tried to think of a reasonable answer but could come up with none. 'Well I guess you're right,' he conceded at last. Of course I was but the problem is that society sees tall as genetic and wide as man-made, and therein lies the lie. Now here's an interesting headline I would like to wave in Mr. Journalist's face. 'Hardwired for Fat: Scientists identify Obesity Gene.'

British and French scientists have identified several variants on a single gene that boost the risk of obesity according to a study published in the British Journal Nature. Previous research has shown that a rare mutation of the same PCSK1 gene can all by itself cause massive gains in weight. In a study of 13,000 European people, mutations of this gene were far more common in obese people. It seems this errant gene produces an enzyme that plays a critical role in converting the hormones that control appetite and regulate energy metabolism. A series of recent discoveries have confirmed these findings and indicate that genetics play a much greater role in weight gain than previously thought. 'By the end of the year,' the researcher continues, 'we will have probably identified a dozen genes that are linked to obesity.' Now while I prefer to pin it on astrology, I'll accept these findings gracefully.

So if we're going to have a fat tax on airlines then I insist on fairness. First we should introduce a height tax so that those obnoxious tall leggy passengers, like Mr. Journalist, will stop poking the back of my seat with their lethal limbs and injuring my spine much more than any wide person would do sitting next to me. While we're at it I'd like to see the introduction of a noise tax so that those parents who think its acceptable for little Brighton to run amok in the aisles screaming at the top of his lungs for the entire twenty hour trip to the outer reaches of Alaska will think again. I want to see hostie Colleen add a noise meter to her tools so she can measure the decibels and charge accordingly.

If you're going to charge, don't discriminate. If you're too fat, too tall, too stupid, too loud, too drunk, too smelly or just downright obnoxious then prepare to pay. All for one and one for all. Not one fat person alone. No way. If it's any consolation there's no end to Ryanair's remarkable initiative.

Now they're in talks with US plane makers Boeing about adapting its aircraft so that some passengers could be placed in 'vertical seating.' 'Beam me up, Scotty!' The airline wants to rip out the traditional seating and install 'a stool or similar for passengers to lean on or sit on. They wouldn't be fully standing,' a spokesman for the airline insists. No, I suspect by the time the plane takes off they will be ricocheting around the aircraft, holding on for grim life. Fortunately the fat ones have more weight to keep them grounded while the thin ones would buzz around the cabin like a bunch of wheezing mosquitoes!

FOOD FOR THOUGHT

I had another revelation today. This time it didn't happen in the jungle in Nepal among the animals but rather surrounded by a flock of tourists sunbaking on the beach in Bali. The enchanted island was at its glorious best with the mystic mountain peaking blue on the horizon, ringed by a halo of fairy floss clouds. Thinking I could be no closer to paradise, I lay back in my deck chair enjoying a delicious fruit cocktail. That's when I saw her, rising up from the ocean like Aphrodite. The most superb woman with the body of a goddess. Like Botticelli's Birth of Venus, she was all curves and ripe flesh, perfectly proportioned.

Struck by her beauty, I stirred from my reclining position and wandered over to have a chat. Her name was Paola and she came from Bulgaria. As it turned out Paola owned several clothing boutiques in Sofia, so it was an opportunity to discuss the issue of size with someone from the other side of the globe. 'Is weight a problem in Bulgaria?' I asked, hoping for a resounding no. Surely not in Eastern Europe.

Instead she confirmed my worst fears. 'Oh yes, size is a very big problem,' Paola replied, looking rather defeated. 'Bulgarian women are naturally a large build but they want to be thin. Many young girls are anorexic and starve so they can fit into stylish clothes. It's mostly the fault of the fashion designers. They design fashions for stick insects.'

There can be no excuse for the damage being done across our world. Women are lined up in China for plastic surgery, to widen their eyelids to appear more Western. Children there do not want an Asian version of Barbie but LA Barbie with big blue eyes and blond hair, long legs and a tiny waist. Some people even have their leg bones sawn off and refitted to be painfully elongated and become taller. This is beauty at its worst as we become plastic people in a scary Barbie world.

Images are presented to us on a daily basis carrying mixed messages that overwhelm our senses and confuse us even more. Some of the worst go unnoticed, affecting us on a subliminal level. At a televised charity concert, Posh Spice asked viewers to contribute funds 'to end world poverty, hunger and starvation.' Am I the only one offended here? When celebrities reduce themselves to a stick-thin size O they cause their fair share of damage in the world, including hunger, starvation and spiritual poverty, by prompting others to follow their lead. Many women who try to copy such examples are reduced to wretched shells of their beautiful selves. What a tragic state of affairs.

Despite all the dire warnings about weight, a new Japanese study has found that being very skinny carries much more risk and is more dangerous than being fat. Apparently *slightly chubby people live the longest,* despite all the advice to the contrary. What's more people who are a little overweight at the age of forty, live six to seven years longer than very thin people whose life expectancy was five years shorter than that of obese people. Skinny people have heightened vulnerability to diseases such as pneumonia and various types of nasty bugs.

Adding credibility to this theory is a number of similar studies which confirm the findings of the Japanese one. One of the latest of these is a twelve year Canadian study that confirmed earlier findings by researchers 'that overweight appears to be protective against mortality, while being thin correlates with higher death risk.' But this is an issue that goes beyond science and even health and becomes a question of what constitutes an expression of beauty and acceptance in our world.

To those persons in the public eye who diminish themselves from their original healthy state and prompt others to follow their lead, this is a wakeup call to develop a social conscience. Renee Zelweiger was exuberant in Brigitte Jones' Diary but shrunk down into skin and bones. Sophie Dahl stood out as a plush super-size model and made many of us feel great. Until she decided to conform and become just another face on the catwalk. Rachel Weisz was yummy in the Mummy and then spoiled it by becoming super lean as did countless other movie stars.

Kelly Osbourne, eccentric Ozzy Osbourne's daughter, had her own distinctive style which she sacrificed in part when she lost over forty pounds and turned from a plump stunning redhead into a regular blond. However I understand her plight and applaud her effort. After therapy to deal with the issues, Kelly confessed, 'When you're a fat girl in Hollywood, it's not fun. You never get looked at the way skinny girls do.' Which raises the question of who actually needs therapy, her or the residents of la la land? The answer is patently clear and it ain't her.

Shame on those tabloids that churn out photos of warped body images, tampering with photos to make stars look 'perfect' or whacking on bulges of cellulite to shock us and humiliate them. Jessica Simpson was on the receiving end of a great deal of media abuse when she was accused of being fat, all while sporting tiny size 4 jeans, well below the national average size. Although she admitted to being hurt, Jessica had the strength to state wisely that beauty should be celebrated in all forms. She went on to make a TV show 'The Price of Beauty' and travelled the world to see what constituted beauty in different countries.

In France she met with the model Isabelle who after being told by one agency that she had to lose over twenty pounds, became anorexic and went on to a near death state of starvation. In a coma three years ago she was not expected to pull through but she survived and went on to create shocking billboard posters of her nude skeletal body declaring, 'No to Anorexia.' The celebrity hair stylist Ken Paves who travelled with Jessica stated that he was embarrassed and ashamed of the beauty industry for the damage it had inflicted on women. Wise words indeed.

An opinion shared by stunning Portia de Rossi, partner of Ellen DeGeneres, who knows better than most the high price one has to pay to reach an unrealistic modeling standard. A woman who exudes both inner and outer beauty, she was cut down in her teens when an agent commented on her saggy butt. She too went on a downward spiral into acute anorexia and after many years of struggle and facing

191

her inner demons she fought her way out and now inspires countless others with her journey as written in her moving book Unbearable Lightness, A Story of Loss and Gain. That just about sums it up.

Life can be harsh and appears to conspire against us from the time we are young. Larger children are never portrayed as heroes or as princesses but more often like ogres, Fiona and Shrek. They are *not* kind-hearted monsters but beautiful and lovely just as they are, although there are few examples to convince them of the fact. Disney studios need to rise to the occasion. They made their first animated film featuring a black princess. Next, how about a realistically sized one to serve as an example of true rather than idealized animated beauty.

When I spoke with a friend, a young man with a liberal outlook about the subject of beauty no matter the shape he stated, 'Yes, there is beauty in imperfection.' I corrected him. Beauty in all its forms *is* perfect. In England a county's choice of a size 12 entrant as their representative in the Miss UK contest drew derisive comments in the press. It appears we still have a long way to go. Israel is far ahead, having held a 'Miss Fat and Beautiful' beauty contest for the past fifteen years. The last winner was a stunning beauty of one hundred and eighty pounds, a far more realistic depiction of a woman with a rich Israeli heritage.

Thankfully a handful of designers have risen to the challenge of creating clothes that go beyond restrictions of size and stereotype. US designer Bradley Bayou, who has dressed Oprah, spoke out against hiring ultra thin models. His own daughter had a six year battle with bulimia and he is an ambassador for the US National Eating Disorder Association. 'Wanting to look like a skeleton is ridiculous,' he states and his style guide 'The Science of Sexy' features women from sizes 4 to 26. Exactly the way it should be, sensuality and style in all its forms.

What a great segment on the program 'The View' when Beyonce appeared with her gracious mother, Tina Knowles. Mum, who has been designing fabulous clothes for her daughters, has branched out with her own label. It was a defining moment to see two sets of models parade on the show in the same garment, one model slim and the other one plump. Both were attractive in their own right. As Tina said, 'whether you're a size 2 or 22 you deserve good fashion.' Co-host curvaceous Sherri Shepherd said, 'Kudos, to you,' obviously aware of the struggle most larger people have to go to through to feel good about themselves. Whoopi Goldberg raised an important topic about how young people are adversely influenced by the media's unhealthy emphasis on body shape. The latest youth survey in Australia revealed that body image was the number one issue that young people were concerned with today. Not bullying, school performance, family. No, body image.

Government and educational initiatives that encourage children to identify their own uniqueness and not fall victim to society's stereotypes are valid and worthwhile. However there must be a careful balance so that too much pressure is not placed on the child that does not fit in to conform to a sporting and dietary regime that does not suit their constitution, interests or temperament. Don't force them to be who they are not or make them feel guilty when they don't measure up.

Films with plump leads are rare but inspiring. Who can forget glorious plump Muriel in Muriel's Wedding? To an Abba tune her bulky thighs stuffed in white satin were unforgettable. On a more serious note the film Why Did I Get Married? showed the ordeal and insecurities of a larger woman abused and put down by her husband. The film Precious was a tale of a downtrodden, big girl who rose above a torrent of abuse and a miserable life to eventually triumph. TV programs like Gray's Anatomy and Glee owe much of their popularity to the fact that they portray all shapes and shades of people as attractive, with all the emotions and intricacies of the human condition.

Abuse takes many forms and one of the most damaging is verbal abuse. Fortunately we refuse to stand for it any longer. This headline dated 28/10/2010 says it all. 'Attack on fatties sparks outrage.' 'A writer for Marie Claire magazine has been forced to issue an apology for writing an online opinion column in which she called overweight people 'aesthetically displeasing.' She also likened them to alcoholics and heroin addicts and compared watching an obese person to the likes of looking at a drunk person stumbling across a bar or a heroin addict slumping in a chair.' Sorry, but has this woman been taking crack?

Doesn't the writer think that larger people have emotions and feelings and are just as beautiful and loving as the rest? Doesn't the writer think? Her comments are terribly ironic considering the term for ultra thin models is heroin chic. Thin, grungy, emaciated and gaunt were all the go in the modeling world and some advertisers believed to be in vogue you had to look as if you had just shot up heroin into your collapsed veins. And they make us out to be the ones with the problem.

The magazine writer, who should think very carefully before transferring idle thought to computer ever again, was referring to a new show on CBS, a comedy sitcom about a bulky couple named Mike and Molly. Foolishly she wrote, 'I'd be grossed out if I had to watch two characters with rolls of fat kissing each other. I'd be grossed out if I had to watch them doing anything.' Apparently the rest of the country has no such reservations as the show was watched by 12.3 million viewers making it the most popular new comedy of the TV season.

There was a massive backlash against the article and it was heartening to see people react with righteous indignation for they had every reason to be offended by her words. Most people have been forced to deal with weight issues at some time and know the frustration involved. If they do not have a problem themselves they know of a family member or friend who has suffered at its hands or if not, are informed and compassionate enough to understand the hurt involved. As a result of the crass comments thousands of outraged readers vowed to cancel their magazine subscriptions, hence the enforced apology.

The admission by the writer of her previous ordeal with anorexia did little to salve the wounds. Having been forced to face her own challenges in the past she should have been far more empathic to other people's struggles. Obviously she has not addressed her own body image issues and still finds any semblance of fat abhorrent. Sad. In terms of her being 'grossed out watching 'fatties' kiss', most people are far more turned off watching a pair of synthetic skinnies locking collagen enhanced lips on the movie screen, their trout pouts fusing into bony gridlock. Or when fashion shows or magazines insist on using stick thin models as their ideal. We're not boys, we're real women! As one fashion photographer quipped after bedding one model too many, 'It was like going to bed with a bicycle.' Most men prefer something softer to hold on to, with a bit of padding to cushion a bumpy ride!

Reality shows are candy wrapped. Dating shows feature a stud who has his pick of a bunch of lithe blond 'beauties', many of whom have the IQ of a retarded rabbit. When Fox TV took a bold step and introduced a reality dating show called 'More to Love' it scored big in the ratings. The winning lady was a stunning dark beauty who was beautiful on all levels and the bachelor was a lucky man to have found her. The problem however with the program is the premise that plus goes with plus. That large people can only attract a large partner.

This is untrue. In the course of my life I've had a number of fulfilling relationships. I married a handsome Sagittarian man in my youth when I was obsessed with the Beatles because he reminded me of Paul McCartney. This was followed by a gentle introverted Pisces, tall and slim, who played the Spanish guitar. Then came my Gemini jungle man who couldn't sit still long enough to be anything but lean. It was love at first sight with my charismatic Libran who was shorter and louder and loved to dance. Then the love of my life thundered in like Zeus, a gorgeous Aquarian with the well honed body of a Greek god and a mind just as sharp. That's just to name a few, so don't believe that plump women are not appealing to handsome, intelligent, virile men. It's a myth. That goes for the men too because women are attracted by the eyes, the sensuous arms, or to the soft, cuddly type like a sweet teddy bear, a loving kind partner or a gentle giant.

In a major step forward Lifetime TV cast a lovely large lady, Brooke Elliott, as the brilliant lawyer in their show 'Drop Dead Diva.' Its debut show attracted 2.8 million viewers which was the highest rating for an original drama series debut on Lifetime. It just goes to show that we've waited a long, long time for a smart plus sized heroine to be portrayed on television, one that we can finally relate to.

To sweeten the mix is an interesting premise that inside the plump smart brunette is a slender blond bimbo just waiting to get out. It appears they both died at exactly the same moment and the petulant blond model zapped back down to earth in the wrong body. Having been deemed a shallow, self centered type who had achieved nothing of consequence during her lifetime the blond scored a zero at heaven's gate. It was hoped that she would pick up a few pointers on inner beauty inside the smart altruistic lawyer's body, who took a bullet for her boss.

The premise of the show becomes dodgy with the expectation that the boyfriend will one day recognize his lost love inside the dumpy brunette, who to my mind is far more attractive. We need to go beyond the crass stereotyping of smart brunette, bimbo blond, cool mean blond, and distinguish the expression of beauty whatever its shape. Beauty is beauty whatever form it takes. Love is love. It involves substance and depth and is multi layered. It is also balanced so that very few of us miss out in the romance stakes. That's what makes the world go round.

There is supreme order in the heavens and a whole lot of divine wisdom. It's man who screws it up and gets it all wrong. The Creator knew exactly what he was doing when he created his universe, and us in it. While we readily accept differences in skin color and racial diversity, eyes slanted or wide and sparkling from brown, blue, violet, green to hazel, all shades of hair from glossy straight black to frizzy brown, raunchy red to sleek blond, tall and short people, freckles, tattoos and even the occasional hairy mole, we still can't wrap our mind around differences in body shape even though it's staring us in the face.

Asians are generally leaner, Scandinavians taller, some born in the Mediterranean are plump while others are slim, many Africans are of a sturdy powerful build, while Pacific Islanders are generally robust and strong. So the differences continue and within these are countless variations, races within races, that guarantee that we are all different and fabulous in our own right. How hard is that to understand or to accept? It's written in the stars, the divine wisdom of the cosmos, that every person is a one of a kind. To add even more diversity and ensure an unparalleled variety in the human race, relationships are no longer defined by borders but rather by attraction, adding a rich melting pot of genes and creating the beautiful 'indigo children' we will all become.

It's the way of the world. Flowers come in magnificent shapes, colors, scents and hues, and we each have our personal favorite. Fruit and veggies are not restricted to stalks of celery and lean bananas and carrots. We love our apples, oranges and fat juicy stone fruit and berries. Birds range from tiny flitting hummingbirds, chubby sparrows to stunning pink flamingos and gangly ostriches. Fish can swim in a swarm of lean sardines which we catch to eat while whales can swallow us up whole. Look once again at the animal kingdom and the fabulous variety it presents, from the tiniest mouse to the towering elephant. It's nature in all its glory just as mankind should be. A fantastic variety.

We are each created as unique beings, part of the universe's supreme plan. The prime target of love is ourselves and we must first recognize our own beauty before anyone else can do so. It should be embodied in our every thought and action so we will radiate splendor. Weight will cease to be an issue when we reconnect with our center. Our body and soul will at last resonate as one and we will be whole.

IT MUST BE LOVE

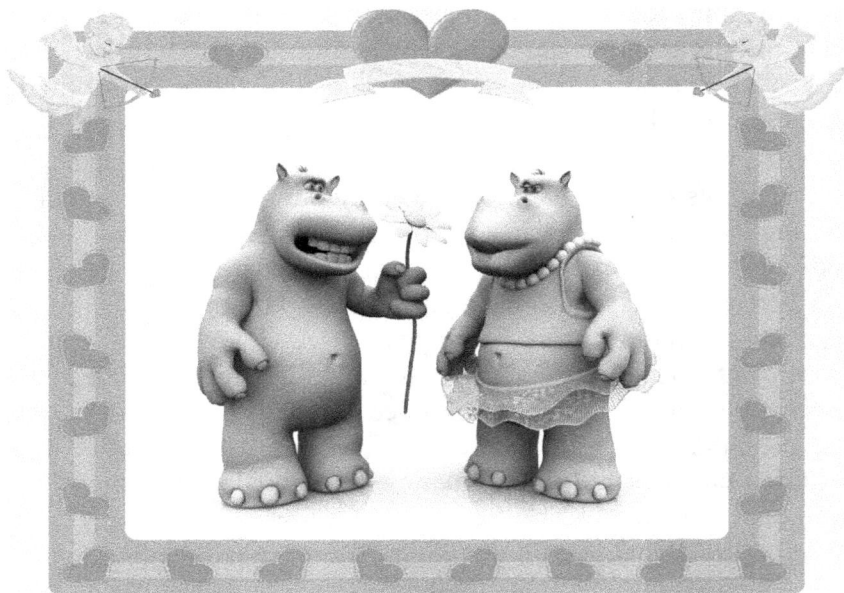

In my twenties I had a lovely friend who was a real sweetie and the cuddly sort. Not fat, just cuddly. She had a special radiance about her, a healthy glow that added to her beauty. She didn't see it at all, that inner spark that shone on the outside and attracted people to her. Instead she succumbed to bulimia and locked herself in the bathroom to purge. Her beautiful curves caved in as she became haggard and drawn.

What I found remarkable was the fact that she attracted a critical Virgo man into her life, a man she was to later marry, who reinforced her poor image of herself. Together they would head off jogging each day and then pumped weights at the gym until they were both totally exhausted from the effort. Despite her strenuous workouts and strict diet regime he always made a point of putting her down, continually commenting on her big bum and how she needed to lose a few pounds.

Compared to her, my behind looked like the back of a bus but I had no problem with it because it provided valuable padding while I sat at my desk writing and my man loved it. I had grown to love my curves and attracted an equally accepting man into my life. As a Libran like myself, my friend was meant to be curvy so when she lost weight she also lost some of her essential beauty and sadly part of her spirit.

A neighbor of mine, an overachieving young Aries woman, also had a critical partner. They both appeared shallow and obsessed with their physical appearance to the detriment of everything else. Each morning she sprinted off to work, miles across the Harbor Bridge, while he drove off in his sports car. She was fit and thin but she was never happy and in the end she became severely anorexic and dried up. Fortunately with therapy she was able to get rid of her obsession, her anorexia, her own self loathing and last of all her demeaning husband.

In the wonderful British movie Shirley Valentine we see just how vital recognition of the self is. Dejected Shirley decides on impulse to go away with a friend on holiday to Greece, in the hope of soaking up the sunshine and finding herself. Unwilling to tell her husband of her plans, she scrawls a message for him on a poster of the Greek islands stuck on the kitchen door. Drawing on her courage she steps onto the plane, leaving behind her boring life in drizzly old England and an even more mundane husband who fails to appreciate her any more. They have fallen into a dreary routine and she has resorted to talking to the wall which provides considerably more stimulation than her husband.

Once in Greece, Shirley relaxes for the first time in years, revels in the white sand and blue seas before falling for the questionable charms of a local man, Costos. One rollicking scene shows the now bubbly, sun kissed Shirley lying on the deck of a sailing ship in the blue waters of the Aegean being made love to by the mad Greek. The boat rocks such is the thrust of their passion and the ocean sighs. In the throes of lovemaking, the mad Greek caresses Shirley's ample body and nibbles at her stretch marks. As you can imagine Shirley is appalled, probably having tried to erase any trace of them away with cooking lard over the past few years or to pound them away with a potato masher.

The mad Greek admonishes her for her prudishness and nibbles some more. 'Shir...ley, Shir...ley,' he croons, in a lovely mellow tone that only a virile Greek can get away with. 'Do not be ashamed of these lines. These are the signposts of your life,' inferring that every groove and mark had its own story to tell. Shirley giggles, unfamiliar with the philosophical ramblings of a wise but crazy Greek. However Shirley is nobody's fool, having been downtrodden for too long to fall for it.

She chuckles to herself and mutters, 'What a load of crap.' Nonetheless she's impressed. Shirley *wants* to hear it because she's been deprived of praise for so long. On this stunning Greek island, Shirley gets a job in a local cafe and happily does her own thing. In so doing she reconnects with herself and once free her spirit glows. She blossoms in the sun and is reborn. Her husband comes to fetch her but she will never go back to her old life until he too is released and learns to appreciate in her what was lost and find himself in the process.

It is essential that Shirley see her own beauty before anybody else can. To do this she needed the help of a wise but mad Greek who was fulfilling his life's purpose. Like Zeus on mighty Olympus, he ravaged a lot of ladies in his quest to make the world a better place and release their inner Hera. True love understands that people change and that their loved one's looks alter over the years, into a more mellow form. Love is not mere physical attraction but awe for the substance that lies beneath the surface. The essence of the person radiates through the eyes and vibrates through their being. That's true love.

If we understand that there are higher truths that bring people together it will take the pressure off the need to conform to a certain shape or look to attract a partner. We have been programmed to believe in a certain ideal of beauty but the reality is much different. Attraction is formed from a complex hierarchy of energetic levels. The most profound comes from past lives where a deep attachment has already formed. If reincarnation is not part of your belief system, allow yourself to be open to the possibility because it explains so much. Couples once happy together may want to reunite or perhaps forbidden lovers may wish to make up for lost time. Nothing can outshine a love that has been forged over centuries, no matter the outer appearance.

Take the love triangle between Prince Charles, Princess Diana and Camilla Parker Bowles for example. Society had trouble accepting the notion of genuine love between Camilla and Prince Charles for a long time. Compared to the lithe, swan like beauty of Princess Diana, Camilla did not meet the traditional concept of beauty. However there may have been a karmic element involved. According to the BBC, 'Camilla inherited the role of royal mistress,' as her great grandmother Alice Keppell was the long time mistress of Prince Charles' great great grandfather, the Prince of Wales. When his mother, Queen Victoria passed away, he ascended to the throne as King Edward 7th.

Mrs. Keppel was the longest serving mistress of the king and remained so until his death. They had a special bond and she was one of the few people who could diffuse the king's many mood swings. Their affair was not a secret and in Edwardian high society bed hopping was acceptable if it was kept discreet. If one can accept the concept of reincarnation, then it's conceivable that Camilla and Charles were once these lovers who were reborn in this lifetime to reunite in an open way. With a bond forged through the years, one that was tolerated but hidden for a very long time, they are now free to declare their love and marry.

When Edward 8th of England met American divorcee Wallis Simpson he was instantly smitten. She did not conform to what was acceptable; either in the beauty stakes or in marital status, but the king's affection for her was unshakeable. She was a Catholic, twice divorced, and even though she was described as a rakish, abrasive woman he was infatuated and showered her with money and jewels.

The king's love for her became a crisis for Britain and although she agreed to stand aside rather than cause a rift in the Empire, the king would not hear of it. Instead he chose to abdicate and in 1936 he handed over his crown to his brother, who became King George VI, during the difficult and challenging times of the Second World War. Despite all the obstacles they faced, Edward and Wallis married and their bond was so strong they remained together until death.

When it is your time, and part of the universal plan, love will happen. That moment of serendipity when you bump into an old friend that you haven't seen for years and it becomes more, or you meet a stranger who takes your breath away. That's when divine providence takes over. It doesn't matter the size of your waist or the designer shoes you wear. If you attract a mate on the basis of such superficial criteria would you want them? Your answer to that question speaks volumes.

The cosmos, universe, creator, God or the Great Almighty is not uncaring or cruel, although at times may appear unreceptive to our needs. It can be frustrating but it may simply not be the right time. Take heart, there is a perfect plan written in the stars. Physical attraction is guaranteed when Venus and Mars connect in a couple's charts. There will be instant chemistry from the moment their eyes meet. You could be the dullest woman of all time, the leanest or the chunkiest, with appalling habits and stubby nails but he'll think you're drop dead gorgeous. She'll want to crawl all over your body and ravage you even though you're plagued with acne or are drunk. It's pure kismet.

There's perfect order in the universe which ensures each of us gets a piece of the action. Some folk may be more blessed than others if they are the flavor of the month, tutti frutti rather than rocky road, but true love will only blossom if there is a soul connection between two people. First, one must be attracted physically. The laws of the universe ensure that each person has their own concept of what constitutes beauty and in so doing balances our chances out.

In a man's chart the placement of Venus indicates what type of woman turns him on, one who oozes sex appeal in his eyes. In a woman's chart, Mars determines who she finds attractive or hot. Of course it's a lot more complicated to come up with a perfect match but let's begin with the basics so you get the gist of the laws of attraction. It's very fair. Some men like girls broad and sassy, others lean and mean, some go for the shy and introverted type while others prefer a sporty or athletic lass to match their latest hatchback car. Let's look more closely at how Venus leaves her mark on our men folk.

Men with a Venus placement in the ample signs of Libra, Cancer, or Pisces will like their women curvy. They are attracted to soft gentle women who make them feel warm and fuzzy. In Aries and Sagittarius they prefer them tall, tanned and athletic. In Aquarius petite with pale skin and somewhat serious or eccentric. And so on. There is a perfect plan in the universe and beauty is definitely a personal preference.

While physical attraction is necessary to first connect two people, all the planets must kick in to ensure a meaningful relationship between them. Venus and Mars ignite the passion, the moon allows you to share emotions and Mercury lets you explain how you feel. Saturn ensures that the relationship lasts and has meaning, while Jupiter makes you learn, laugh and feel happy together. Uranus gives it excitement, Pluto depth and Neptune the spiritual connection of a true soul mate.

The process is further complicated because countries as well as people have their own horoscope. It determines the nation's character, its thought processes, values and principles. Depending on the position of Venus, it also influences the country's ideal of beauty. The fourth of July is the date the United States celebrates its independence. It's a Cancerian nation, with four planets in the sign, making it cardinal and determined. The Sun, Mercury, Venus and Jupiter combined make a formidable collection and ensure America takes on a 'mothering' role in the world. Venus joined to abundant Jupiter in the sign of Cancer means the people like their food, in big portions. This makes for a nation of large people and an attraction to abundance in all its forms.

Australia's national day on January 26th makes it a progressive Aquarian country. In 1901 when it was declared a federation there was a glut of planets in Sagittarius, the sign that rules sport. Hence the national obsession with it. Not only do people love to play sport but they're also very good at it. Venus is also positioned in the sign of Sagittarius, so the ideal female is tall, leggy and preferably blond. A woman who is active, healthy and boundless like Elle Macpherson or Jennifer Hawkins, a previous Miss Universe. These ladies belong windswept and languishing on a long stretch of beach. Sagittarian energy is male orientated, hence Aussie men are into watching football or cricket with their buddies and woman are more their mates rather that the loves of the lives. They are not the real romantic sort.

If you're wondering where you belong and where you will meet the love of your life then let me introduce you to Astrocartography. It transposes your birthchart onto a world map. In so doing a maze of connections are uncovered. Where your planetary lines fall shows your relationship with different places in the world and their effect on you.

My Sun, Neptune line dissect exactly over Bali. The island is a small dot on a world map yet it became my home after a one week holiday turned into an incredible twenty year love affair. Speaking of love, my Venus line which shows the optimum place for romance, sprawls right across the Pacific Ocean. It's difficult to make contact with any men who might be sailing past or scuba diving below the surface so it's rather frustrating. However each time I go on a cruise in the Pacific I'm involved in some hot and heavy romance and watch the sparks fly when I hit Noumea. All those lovely, romantic Frenchmen.

It's obvious the Pacific islands have a bountiful Venus position which explains their admiration for big ladies. When I got off the plane for a one night layover in Guam, a small island in the Pacific, I couldn't believe my luck. Obviously my Venus line extended as far as its shores. In the course of a day I was asked out on more dates than I ever had in Australia over the span of thirty years! All this in my golden years. How frustrating to suddenly grasp exactly what you'd been missing.

When I arrived in Hawaii it got even better. Men left notes under my hotel room door and were chatting me up in the elevator. Mars was heating up and I had struck Venus gold. I found the men as desirable as they found me. But why had it taken a lifetime to discover that I was attractive to the opposite sex? All because I had grown up in the 'wrong' place for romance. Simply put, I didn't fit in to my country's norm of what constituted the ideal woman. Not to say that there weren't men who stepped outside the definition but they were few in number.

While in Hawaii I was fortunate to see a street parade to honor their late king. It was a colorful cavalcade, with floral floats and marching bands. One of the highlights of the parade was the presence of the 'Queens' of the eight Hawaiian islands. Each rode by on a horse surrounded by attendants. One rode by on a grey steed with golden flowers in her hair and a lavish yellow cloak. Another sat proudly on a white horse all decked out in pink blossoms while another straddled a black horse resplendent in a lei of red hibiscus. One regal lady was decked out in green foliage, another wore a mauve feathered gown.

Each queen was stunning in her own right. They were statuesque, grand women who embodied the beauty of their island. Their proud bearing reflected their confidence in their heritage and their magnetic aura marked them out as special. This was beauty at its best. One study concluded that people of the Pacific islands were the happiest on earth. Island people are not only big in body but in spirit too only going to prove that big *is* beautiful. What's more they're proud of it.

Western society is a lot shallower and is ruled by vanity. Vanity is defined as the 'excessive belief in one's attractiveness to self and others.' While it's a positive thing to feel good about ourselves it's another to concentrate on our looks to our own detriment. In religion, vanity was considered one of the seven deadly sins because it was seen as a rejection of God in favor of one's own image. Pride is considered the original and most serious of the deadly sins, beating out lust, sloth, envy and wrath. Even greed and gluttony pale in comparison.

Vanity was the reason Lucifer was cast out of Heaven. The Archangel wanted to make his throne higher than the clouds over earth where he could preside above all others and resemble 'the power on high.' Unfortunately his lofty ambitions proved to be his undoing, as they often do, and as we all know 'pride comes before the fall.' Lucifer was downgraded to Satan and did his penance doing time in hell.

Lucifer is the name given to the Morning Star which is the planet Venus in its dawn appearance. Venus outshines both Saturn and Jupiter but as an 'inner planet' its appearance is brief and it soon disappears from the night sky. Which only goes to illustrate how beauty is both transient and illusory and viewed differently in each place.

The epitome of vanity was Narcissus, an extremely attractive but not so bright Greek lad who fell in love with his own reflection in a pool of water. He was so taken with his own image he didn't realize he was staring at himself. It was only when he went to kiss his reflection that reality dawned on him. In anguish he took a sword and killed himself and in sadness his body turned into a flower, the Narcissus.

In the Roman version of the story, a forest nymph Echo fell in love with the handsome youth while he was hunting in the woods. Echo was too shy to approach him but when he heard her footsteps, he shouted, 'Who's there?' She repeated his words, and on it went until he challenged her to show herself and she rushed out to embrace him.

The vain youth pulled away from her and cruelly told her to leave him alone. Echo was heartbroken and spent the rest of her time alone and despondent in forest glens, pining for the love she never knew until only her voice remained. Thirsty, Narcissus went to drink from a stream but fearing that he would destroy his own reflection, he died from thirst while staring longingly at himself. Then out popped a flower.

Learn from these stories and from songs like, 'You're so vain' and 'Never make a pretty woman your wife,' because basically you'll regret it for the rest of your life. To be consumed with one's appearance and how you compare to others, to the point that you wish to become like them to the detriment of yourself, is not only foolish but also the worst form of vanity. Be natural and gracefully accept your own beauty.

What I suggest you do is stare at yourself in a lake or a mirror until you can see the real person that lies within the depths of your soul. You don't want to look down and see a modified version of yourself or an artificial one that society has created. Friedrich Nietzsche wrote that 'vanity is the fear of appearing original.' So in order not to be vain be original instead. Discover who you are and what makes you unique and you will attract others to you. You don't have to search the world for that special someone because they might just wash up onto your shores. Be open to the possibility and anything can happen and probably will.

The last word goes to a charming Sydney bus driver. Bless him. In the midst of peak hour traffic and the usual crush of sinewy, strained office workers who were shoving me aside, he gazed at me when I climbed on board and asked if I had any concessions. When I said no, he replied, 'If there was a concession for beauty, you'd ride for free.'

So if you want a wonderful ride through life then recognize your own particular brand of beauty without someone else having to remind you of it, although that's always a bonus! It's not so much vanity or conceit but rather an appreciation of your natural being which embodies the spirit of creation. You are beautiful just as you were created to be, like the sun, the moon and the stars. If you want to shimmer just as brightly and be the center of your universe then celebrate who you are. Beauty is a radiance, an essence that shines from within to resonate on the outside. Fan your inner flame until it glows and remember a big blaze burns brighter and the flames linger longer. Whatever your shape you are the essence of love and beauty, you only have to believe it.

If you do then so will the rest of the world.

www.ingramcontent.com/pod-product-compliance
Lightning Source LLC
Chambersburg PA
CBHW072133270326
41931CB00010B/1746